SOME MUST WATCH
WHILE SOME MUST SLEEP

SOME MUST WATCH WHILE SOME MUST SLEEP

William C. Dement
STANFORD UNIVERSITY

W. H. FREEMAN AND COMPANY
San Francisco

Library of Congress Cataloging in Publication Data

Dement, William Charles, 1928-
    Some must watch while some must sleep.

    Reprint of the 1972 ed. published by Stanford Alumni
Association, Stanford, Calif., in series:
The Portable Stanford
        Bibliography: p.
        1. Sleep.   2. Dreams.   I. Title.
[QP425.D44 1974]   612'.821   74-7334
ISBN 0-7167-0769-1
ISBN 0-7167-0768-3 (pbk.)

Printed in the United States of America

9   8   7   6   5   4

This book was published
originally as a part of
The Portable Stanford,
a series of books published by
the Stanford Alumni Association.

CONTENTS

ILLUSTRATIONS

Illustrations throughout this book are from the work of Pablo Picasso. The theme of "the sleeper watched" was suggested by Dr. Dement, and is largely drawn from the article "Sleep Watchers," by Leo Steinberg, *Life*, Dec. 27, 1968. Many of the illustrations in this book appeared in that article. Some illustrations (pages 10-11, 29, 88-89) are from *L'Oeuvre Gravé de Picasso*, published by Clairefontaine at Lausanne, Switzerland, 1955. We are grateful to Cahiers d'Art, Paris, France, publishers of the massive multivolume *Picasso*, by Christian Zervos, for permission to reproduce the drawings on the cover and on pages xvi, 20, 34, 54, 67, 94, and 103.

Other illustrations from the work of Picasso:

PAGE 17   *Meditation*, late 1904. Watercolor and pen, 13⅝″ × 16⅛″. Collection, Mrs. Bertram Smith, New York.

PAGES 42-43   *Vigil*, 1936. Etching, 9⅝₁₆″ × 11¹¹⁄₁₆″. Collection, The Museum of Modern Art, New York. Purchase.

PAGE 49   *The Dream*, 1952. Collection, Dr. A. Kladetzky-Haubrich, Cologne.

PAGES 60-61   *Faun and Sleeping Woman*, 1936. Etching and aquatint, 12⁷⁄₁₆″ × 16⁷⁄₁₆″. Collection, The Museum of Modern Art, New York. Purchase.

PAGE 72   *Sleeping Nude*, 1904. Collection, Jacques Helft, Paris.

PAGE 84   *Minotaur and Woman*, 1933. Drypoint, printed in black, 11⅝″ × 14⅜″. Collection, The Museum of Modern Art, New York. Purchase.

The sleep research figures on pages 106, 107, 109, 110, 111, and 114 are by Jim M'Guinness.

The photographs on pages 115 and 120-121 were provided by Dr. Dement.

PREFACE

When I agreed to write a book about sleep and dream research at the behest of the Stanford University Alumni Association, I hoped to make my account as fascinating and exciting as the research itself has been. Admittedly, the average person would not, at first blush, pick watching people sleep as the most apparent theme for a spine-tingling scientific adventure thriller. However, there is a subtle sense of awe and mystery surrounding the "short death" we call sleep to which people who reflect for a moment almost always respond. I think these feelings must have captured Pablo Picasso's imagination, because *the sleeper watched* was a frequent theme in his drawings, some of which we are privileged to include in the book. Another theme that must have endlessly intrigued him is the eternal question, "But does she dream of me?"

During the present writing, I was often in conflict between the desire to be comprehensive, authoritative, utterly correct, and so forth, and the simple urge to say something that would be remembered. With regard to the latter, I have been strongly influenced by a book that is even slimmer than this one, entitled *1066 and All That*, written in 1931 by W. C. Sellar and R. J. Yeatman. At this point I cannot resist repeating an anecdote that has become a traditional part of the introductory lecture in my course on sleep and dreams for more than eight hundred undergraduates each year. Sellar and Yeatman firmly state that "history is what you can remember." They claim that the average Englishman can remember only about two dates in history, one of which is almost always the Battle of Hastings. The first time I taught the sleep and dream course, I described this remarkable thesis on history and memory and suggested to the students that if the average Englishman could remember little more than the date 1066, I could hardly expect them to remember the myriad details contained in thousands of publications on sleep and dreams. I would therefore, I said, undertake a somewhat different pedagogic style and emphasize principles, particularly A Few Important Principles, that I would expect them to remember for the remainder of their lives. I further suggested that although a future *Memorable Introduction to Sleep Research* might be a very slim volume, we would all know what was in it. Throughout the ensuing semester, I underscored verbally things that the students "should always remember," such as "there are two entirely different kinds of sleep and their names are REM and NREM," "sleeping pills cause insomnia," and so forth. At the end of the semester, well satisfied with myself and my pedagogic philosophy, I gave a multiple-choice examination, but, for the last question, I asked, "write one thing from the course that you will surely remember for the rest of your life." Nearly all the students wrote "1066." To this day, I am not sure whether they were telling me something very profound about the educational process, or whether their response was just an extremely well-executed put-on.

Whether or not I have succeeded in making this book fascinating, I do feel that my book is a satisfactory and authoritative introduction to the sleep field, readable in an evening or two without inducing drowsiness. At the end, the reader will have some awareness of the major problems of sleep research and the overall complexity of sleep and dream processes as well as a few ways in which knowledge of sleep might be personally helpful. If the book stimulates a desire for further exploration, the Reader's Guide at the end of the book contains a fairly substantial number of suggestions for additional reading.

Even with the "1066" philosophy, it was an agonizing task to meet the Stanford Alumni Association's strong mandate for brevity. How to make a point without detailing the endless exceptions and qualifications that scientific tradition requires? There are literally hundreds of dedicated, hard-working sleep researchers, past and present, who have contributed to the mass of facts and speculations in the field. Inevitably, a number of investigators and important research findings did not receive the attention they deserve, and for this I apologize. In addition, I wanted this account to be a somewhat more personal statement than is conventionally the case in an elementary text and have accordingly perhaps overemphasized work done at the Stanford laboratories. In doing so, however, I feel I have been able to convey more about why the work is so intriguing. After more than twenty years of sleep research, I remain undaunted.

Deciding about a title was also a major obstacle. Nearly everyone I consulted on the Stanford faculty thought it should be *Everything You Always Wanted to Know About Sleep,** but as I have already pointed out, the book is not that comprehensive. My students felt that it should be *REM Sleep and All That.* An obvious choice was the well-known quotation, "To sleep, perchance to dream" from *Hamlet* (Act III, Scene I), but another quotation, also from *Hamlet* (Act III, Scene II), finally just could not be resisted. It hits the bull's-eye dead-center as an expression of the sleep researcher's lonely, life-disrupting hours of work, and it is Literary on top of that.

* *But Were Too Tired to Ask.*

The book is intended primarily for students and other persons who have had no prior education in the area of sleep and dream research. It may be particularly useful as supplementary reading in psychology, biology, or medical courses where material pertaining to sleep and dreams is briefly covered. I have used the original Portable Stanford edition quite happily as the basic text in my course and as supplementary reading for practicing physicians in postgraduate medical courses on the diagnosis and treatment of sleep disorders. I also gave copies of the book to many of my friends and relatives for Christmas. They did not complain.

I have been aided by many people in preparing this book and in the research that is behind it. My research is supported by NIMH Grant MH-13860, NASA Grant NGR 05-020-168, and Research Career Development Award MH 5804 from the U.S. Public Health Service. My associates in the Stanford University Sleep Disorders Clinic and Laboratories made the book possible by their forbearance and their willingness to assume some of my daily responsibilities for a time. Jeanne Kennedy prepared the index and glossary for the present edition of the book. A special thanks is due to Mary Carskadon, who worked with me from the first stage of the manuscript, and without whose constant assistance the book might never have emerged from the dark of night. I wish also to acknowledge my friend and teacher, Nathaniel Kleitman, the first source of many of the ideas and findings described herein. My wife, Pat, was a constant source of spiritual inspiration. Finally, we were aided and goaded by members of the Stanford Alumni Association staff.

Stanford, California   *William C. Dement*
April 1974

SOME MUST WATCH
WHILE SOME MUST SLEEP

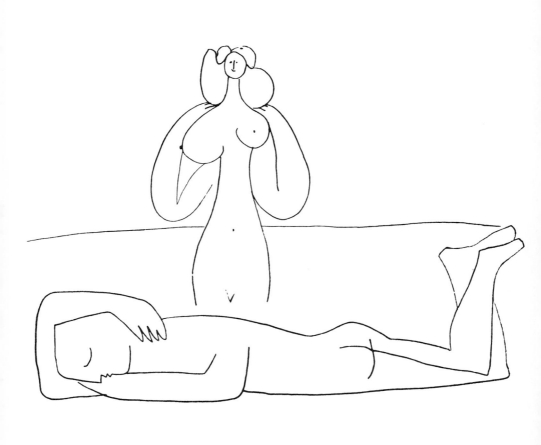

CHAPTER ONE

THE MYSTERY OF SLEEP

WHAT IS IT THAT LURES us each night from our work, our games, our loved ones, into the solitary world of sleep? Driving late one cloudy night in the back country east of Lake Tahoe, my thoughts drifted to this problem. I tried to comprehend the unimaginable gulf between the present and life some million years ago—before man could control fire. How unthinkingly we accept our cities, electric lights, automobiles, our technological miracles! I tried to recall if I had ever been away from all this, somewhere in total darkness where I would have experienced the solitude that must have been known to our distant ancestors. As I mused, I realized that I might be in such a place at that very moment. On an impulse, I turned off the blacktop onto a dirt road and drove perhaps five miles along this winding path. There was no moon, no stars; but for the headlights of my car picking up bits of reality in the vast spread of darkness, I would have felt totally suspended in time and space.

At a wide place in the road, I stopped the car, turned off the lights and the motor, and got out. My hand could feel the cold metal of the car, but I could see nothing. I had walked only a few paces when a wave of apprehension enveloped me. Suppose I got lost? Suppose I became disoriented and could not find my way back to the car? My foreboding increased with each additional step until, in a surge of panic, I turned and started back. But where was the car? How far had I come?

Now the utter darkness, the pitch blackness of the night, filled me with a kind of primordial dread and horror. Groping and stumbling, I managed to locate the car before I became entirely paralyzed by fright. As I climbed back into my warm, safe, familiar automobile, I realized with new insight that night was once man's enemy. The sleep process carried with it a gentle protection from the psychic terrors spawned in the long hours of unrelieved blackness.

Perhaps family life itself originated from the need to sleep and to cluster for protection while in this state. Because sleep occurs during the dark hours when man is least able to cope with his environment, and because man asleep is not alert to the dangers of the outer world, sleep is a state of vulnerability. It is necessary to seek a place of refuge in which to sleep. A troop of baboons has its tree, the wolf has its den; primitive man had his cave or his hut, and we have our bedrooms. Having constructed a safe place to sleep, man is able to use the word "home."

On the lighter side, sleep has also manifested an economic effect in paraphernalia ranging from pillows and pajamas to eiderdown sleeping bags and campers on wheels. Consider the bed. From a simple animal hide or a pile of leaves on a dirt floor, the bed has grown to a box spring and mattress, and now to a water-filled balloon; twin-size, double, queen, king, and room-size; rectangular, square, heart-shaped, or amorphous. The business of lodging travelers has grown from the scattered wayside inns of medieval Europe to thousands of hotels and motels all over the world.

The anthropological and sociological implications of sleep are vast and complex. Yet down through the centuries, while scientists have probed and analyzed man's every waking moment, they apparently dismissed sleep as a time of rest and quiet when absolutely nothing was happening. Those who did pay attention to sleep did so because of its function as the springboard for dreams.

Dreams have enjoyed historic, personal, and religious significance for as long as recorded time. Preserved Babylonian and Assyrian clay tablets, recording dreams and their interpretations, date back to 5000 B.C. Egyptians erected temples to Serapis, god of dreams, where people would sleep in the hope of inducing fortuitous dreams. Dreams and visions are found in at least seventy passages of the Bible, and are discussed in four chapters of the Talmud. For some primitive cultures, dreams were extensions of reality. A chief in equatorial Africa once dreamed he had visited England. When he awakened, he ordered a wardrobe of European clothes; appearing in them, he was congratulated by his friends for having made the trip. When a Cherokee Indian dreamed of a snake bite, he was treated for it. The East Indians categorized good and bad dreams in the sacred *Vedas* written before 1000 B.C. Ancient Chinese belief held that the soul was involved in dreams and could wander from the body when the person was asleep; hence, the sleeper was never hastily aroused. Dreams have spurred military forays, changed political decisions, and led to creative accomplishments. Yet, until sleep was scientifically studied, the occasion, frequency, and stimuli of dreams were not known.

The Need for Sleep

The scientific study of sleep has become intense in recent years, so that today the amount of work being done in sleep laboratories all over the world is awesome. This investigation is resulting in almost daily modification of hypotheses and opinions about various issues in the sleep research field. There is encouraging progress toward answers to the great puzzles: Do we really need to sleep? How much sleep do we need? Why do we sleep? Why do we dream? What is "the stuff that dreams are made of"?

Yet the closer we come to answering these and other questions, the more astounded we are at the richness and variety of our sleeping life. Is it really possible that every night each of us is effectively paralyzed for nearly two hours? How is it that we can experience—see, hear, feel, taste, smell—a whole world of events while we lie quietly in our beds? The sleep abnormalities we have studied are in some ways even more amazing. There are certain individuals who are unable to breathe and sleep at the same time. Others suffer the paralysis of dreaming when they are wide awake.

A discussion of these and other findings will follow, but first I would like to take up the question most frequently asked of a sleep researcher: "How much sleep do I need?"

It would be pleasant to be able to give a brisk, authoritative reply, but we're unable to do that because our research has not yet. answered the even more basic question, "Do we really need to sleep at all?" Furthermore, a real beginning on this question is almost impossible because we do not know what it is that sleep accomplishes at the biochemical level. One way of answering the question of whether or not at least some sleep is an absolute necessity would be to locate a person who never sleeps and yet is healthy and alert at all times. Although a number of claims have been made, they have quickly faded under the cold glare of round-the-clock scientific observation. The existence of even one such person has yet to be documented and I have serious doubts that it ever will be.

At the present time, the main approach to the question of how much sleep is needed is to look at individual differences and to assess the effects of sleep deprivation. A generation ago our hygiene books told us that everybody "needs" eight hours of sleep each night. The fallacy of that rule was demonstrated at our Stanford Sleep Laboratory nine years ago by someone who was living right in our own backyard. He was the late Professor B. Q. Morgan, chairman of Stanford's Department of Germanic Languages for many years and a renowned international scholar.

Professor Morgan told us that it had been his custom to sleep six to eight hours each night until he went to Germany on a fellowship at the age of twenty-three. The change in his sleep habits occurred with unexplained suddenness. One night he went to bed at his usual time of ten o'clock, but woke up at two and could not go back to sleep. He thought little of it, until the next night when, in spite of the same ten o'clock bedtime, he again wakened at two. This time, out of sheer boredom, he lit his candle, and resumed the studies he had discontinued at bedtime. This four-hour sleep pattern continued for the rest of his life—and the professor was quite pleased about it. It did not make him sleepy during the day, and it enabled him to be enormously productive in his academic life. In his retirement years, he continued to waken early, and often stayed in bed passing the time in some useful pursuit such as knitting. He commented that nearly every one of his many friends owned at least one afghan that had been produced entirely before sunrise.

Professor Morgan was kind enough to sleep in our laboratory for five consecutive nights during his eightieth year and to allow one of our staff to accompany him during each of the following days. In this way, we established the indisputable fact that slightly less than four hours was indeed all the "rest" he needed to maintain his amazingly active daytime schedule.

The record for verified short sleep is held by two gentlemen from Australia, ages fifty-four and thirty, who were recorded for seven consecutive nights by Ian Oswald and Raymond Jones. Both were healthy and required less than three hours of sleep a night.

Although there is probably an optimal amount of sleep for each individual, this amount changes from time to time. One of the most common—and most dramatic—changes often occurs during pregnancy, probably due to hormonal effects. I asked several women to keep sleep diaries before, during, and after pregnancy and discovered that during pregnancy there was an increase of approximately two hours in mean daily sleep time.

Years ago, the federal government issued a publication implying that newborn babies "ought to" sleep at least twenty-one hours a day. Besides worrying a lot of mothers whose otherwise normal infants were clearly not sleeping this much, the misinformation goaded Nathaniel Kleitman, dean of American sleep researchers, into conducting a systematic study of neonatal sleep which showed that the *average* sleep time for the newborn is sixteen hours. Of course, some infants slept a great deal less. My own daughter Cathy, whose sleep I carefully tabulated during her first several months, slept about five and one-half hours a day. Unfortunately, for my wife's peace of mind, she spent quite a few of those many waking hours howling at the top of her lungs. Now, at age fourteen (I hasten to add), she sleeps about nine hours a night and has a very pleasant disposition.

The accumulated experience of our sleep laboratory indicates that sixteen-year-olds tend to sleep between ten and eleven hours; college graduate students usually sleep about eight hours.

In addition to the changes that accompany maturation, there are various adaptations to the demands of the environment. I have a sleep diary from one student who slept an average of ten hours a night during the summer but only seven hours and ten minutes a night during the school year. Apparently it is not impossible for a sleep-deprived individual to sleep eighteen hours out of a twenty-four-hour period. But in my own twenty years of experience in sleep research, the longest sleep without prior deprivation that I have observed was seventeen hours—and this individual was able to sleep only five hours the next night.

The classic, though perhaps apocryphal, example of short sleep is Salvador Dali's nap. Dali puts a tin plate on the floor, then sits in a chair beside it; holding a spoon over the plate he relaxes into a doze. At the precise moment of sleep onset the spoon slips from his fingers, clatters onto the plate, and he is snapped awake. Dali claims he is completely refreshed by the sleep that accumulates between the time the spoon leaves his hand and the time it hits the plate.

Sleep Deprivation

The first experiments on the effects of depriving animals of sleep were performed in 1894 by Marie de Manaceine, who found that puppies died when kept awake for four to six days. Other investigators did similar studies and found abnormalities in the animals' brains at autopsy. Nathaniel Kleitman was the first to use control animals who shared exactly the same environment but were allowed to sleep. He found that similar abnormalities were also present in the brains of the control animals. The autopsy revealed nothing that showed the effects of sleep loss or explained why the animals died during the period of sleep deprivation.

The first sleep deprivation study on man was made in 1896 by G. T. W. Patrick and J. A. Gilbert, who kept three young subjects awake for ninety hours and submitted them to a variety of physiological and psychological tests. Unfortunately, the only baseline measurement was the performance of the subjects after the sleep period that terminated the long vigil. Although the experiment was performed only once, there was a certain consistency in the results obtained in the three subjects. There were decreases in sensory acuity, quickness of reaction, motor speed, and memorizing ability. The other significant observations were visual hallucination in one subject and a gradual decrease in body temperature, although the twenty-four-hour temperature curve was preserved. The subjects actually gained weight during the experiment and seemed to be completely restored to normal following twelve hours of sleep at the end of the ninety-hour period.

It has always been questioned whether it is sleep *per se* that makes the crucial difference in the way we feel the next morning, or if it is being in bed, being in the dark, or simply rest. Some people have suggested that the only way a normally impatient human could ever achieve eight continuous hours of good rest is by sleeping. These considerations were in Nathaniel Kleitman's mind when he began his sleep deprivation experiments on human subjects in 1922. His plan was to maintain the routine of living in absolutely everything but sleep. The subjects would undress and go to bed at the usual time but were supposed to stay awake throughout the night while lying quietly in bed. These studies antedated nighttime radio or LP phonographs so the long hours struggling to remain awake in bed in the dark must have been quite a chore. According to Kleitman, complete wakefulness could sometimes be achieved during the first night, but he quickly realized that it was entirely impossible during the second. In order to stay awake the subjects had to engage in some kind of muscular activity, even if it was only talking. Kleitman had arrived at the first paradox of sleep-deprivation studies: the impossibility of separating the effect of sleep loss from the effect of almost uninterrupted muscular activity. He summed up his observations of the behavior of sleep-deprived subjects:

> While there were differences in the subjective experiences of the many sleep evading persons, there were several features common to most. . . . during the first night the subject did not feel very tired or sleepy. He could read or study or do laboratory work without much attention from the watcher, but

usually felt an attack of drowsiness between 3 a.m. and 6 a.m. The drowsiness was accompanied by an unpleasant itching of the eyes. Next morning the subject felt well except for a slight malaise which always appeared on sitting down and resting for any length of time. However, if he occupied himself with his ordinary tasks, he was likely to forget having spent a sleepless night. During the second night the individual's condition was entirely different. His eyes not only itched but felt dry, and he could abolish that sensation only by closing his eyes, which made it extremely hard to remain fully awake even if walking. Reading or study was next to impossible because sitting quietly was conducive to even greater sleepiness. As during the first night, there came a two- to three-hour period in the early hours of the morning when the desire for sleep was almost overpowering. At this time the subject often saw double. Later in the morning the sleepiness diminished once more, and the subject could perform routine laboratory work as usual. It was not safe for him to sit down, however, without the danger of falling asleep, particularly if he attended lectures. Attempting to take down lecture notes usually resulted in failure. . . . All efforts could be sustained for only a short time. An example of this failure was the repeated inability of the subject to count his own pulse for as long as a minute. After counting to fifteen or twenty he invariably lost track of the numbers and would find himself dozing off. The third night resembled the second, and the fourth day was like the third. For this reason we adopted, as a common procedure, a waking period of sixty-two to sixty-five hours. At the end of that time the individual was as sleepy as he was likely to be. Those who continued to stay awake experienced the wavelike increase and decrease in sleepiness with the greatest drowsiness at about the same time every night. (In N. Kleitman, *Sleep and Wakefulness*, Revised and Enlarged Edition, Chicago: University of Chicago Press, 1963.)

Kleitman was one of the first to point out that a severely sleep-deprived subject could pass almost any test with flying colors if such tests were relatively brief. Impairment appeared only during sustained repetitive tasks. Of course, motivation is also very important, and sleep-deprived subjects have great difficulty if they are not sufficiently motivated.

In the 1950s interest in sleep loss reached an all-time peak when it became widely known that experienced inquisitors in police states were using sleep deprivation to induce personality disorders. Such inquisitors were well aware that enforced wakefulness, when combined with emotional turmoil and social isolation, might lead to psychotic behavior in susceptible subjects. A leading authority on psychosis induced by sleep deprivation is Dr. Louis Jolyan West, now chairman of psychiatry at UCLA. Dr. West had extensive experience with American flyers who were captured by the Communists during the Korean conflict and subjected to forceful interrogation. A substantial percentage of these men had signed false confessions stating that they had been engaged in germ warfare. According to Dr. West, some of these confessions were extracted from men who were unquestionably psychotic at the time.

In 1959, I joined Dr. West and his colleagues in observing a New York disk jockey named Peter Tripp, who stayed awake for 200 consecutive hours to raise money for the March of Dimes. Tripp made a daily broadcast from a glass booth on Times Square where crowds could watch him. He was spritely and entertaining, though toward the end of the 200-hour period he began to show impaired performance in the form of slurred or inappropriate speech. In the last days of the marathon, however, a dramatic change occurred. The disk jockey developed an acute paranoid psychosis during the nighttime hours, accompanied at times by auditory hallucinations. He believed that unknown adversaries were attempting to slip drugs into his food and beverages in order to put him to sleep. West and his colleagues described Tripp's mental state as "nocturnal psychosis." Whether or not there was any impairment of his performance abilities on tests at this time could not be determined because he refused to cooperate with the testers during his moments of intense suspicion.

Tripp's condition was not entirely unique. While working in Kleitman's laboratory, I occasionally stayed up forty-eight consecutive hours. (I was a medical student at the time.) During such periods I sometimes became mildly suspicious that my roommates were hostile and were plotting against me. I would say to myself reassuringly, "There is no real reason to feel this way. I know this is ridiculous—it's due to sleep deprivation." Yet the paranoia and the knowledge that it was paranoia existed side by side and did not go away until I had made up my sleep loss.

The Case of Randy Gardner

In 1965, the Stanford group was involved in a sleep deprivation experiment that seriously undermined the notion that unduly prolonged wakefulness could lead to impairment, and particularly that psychosis would be the inevitable result. In January of that year, I chanced to read in the newspapers that a San Diego youth, Randy Gardner, had successfully completed about eighty hours of a planned 264-hour vigil in a high school science fair project aimed at establishing the world's record for prolonged wakefulness. At that time the Guinness Book of World Records listed the record as 260 hours, although real documentation was lacking.

Seeing an opportunity to study prolonged sleep deprivation again, I recruited my colleague, Dr. George Gulevich, now head of the Psychiatric Inpatient Service at Stanford, to accompany me to San Diego with a portable electroencephalograph. The boy's parents welcomed our professional assistance because they were anxious about the consequences of the experiment. Until that time the experiment had been conducted by Randy himself with two of his schoolmates. Although his friends admitted it was not easy to keep him awake in the middle of the night, they testified that he had absolutely not been allowed to sleep. Our main concerns were to verify the lack of sleep and to supplement the inexperienced monitoring of the schoolboys.

Randy, who was seventeen, was a slim boy in excellent physical condition. He was cooperative and friendly throughout, although in the middle of the night when he grew drowsy and wanted to rest his eyes he would object strenuously because we would not allow him to close his lids for any prolonged period of time. As the vigil wore on and impressive durations accumulated, the nation's press and TV became more and more involved until the whole affair began to resemble a circus. This was certainly very stimulating to the young lad and probably aided him in his ability to remain awake. In general, the daytime was relatively easy, but at night we were driven to increasingly heroic measures to help Randy resist sleepiness and to bolster his flagging motivation.

I have two very vivid memories from this study. The first is of spending several hours after 3 a.m. on the last night in a penny arcade where Randy and I competed in about one hundred games on a baseball machine. Randy won every game—which attests to his lack of physical or psychomotor impairment. The second is that, having sacrificed a good deal of sleep myself, I carelessly turned the car into a one-way street the wrong way, and immediately attracted the attention of a policeman. Because of the unusual circumstances, I forgot about the ticket until six months later when a warrant was issued for my arrest. It cost me $86 to redeem myself.

At the end of the long vigil, before going to bed, Randy held a press conference in which the three major TV networks and reporters from papers all over the United States participated. Randy conducted him-

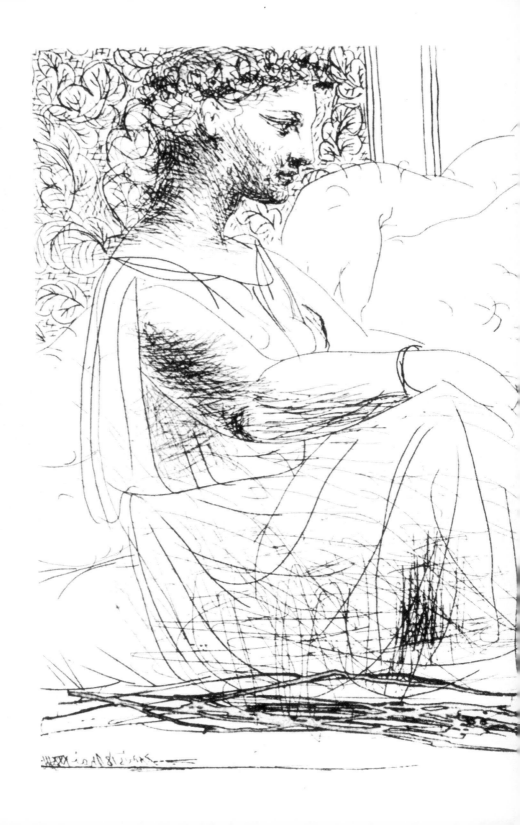

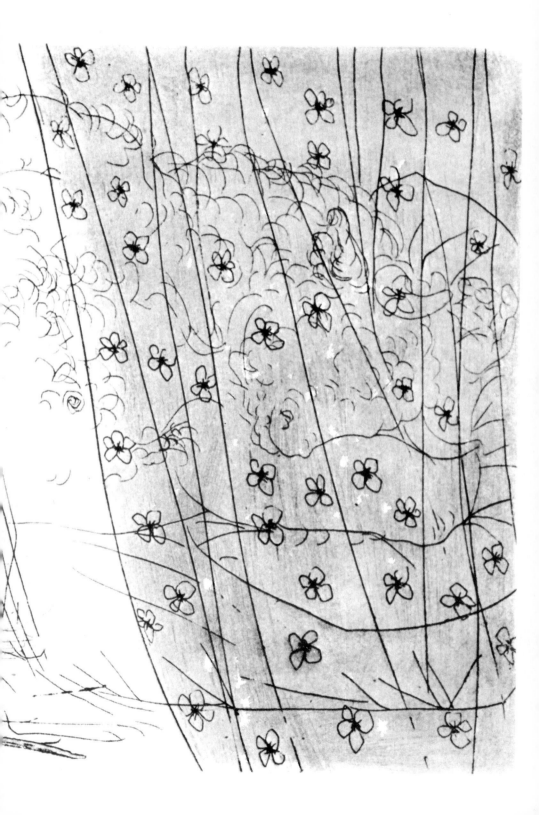

self in an absolutely impeccable fashion. Asked how he was able to stay awake for eleven days, he answered lightly, "It's just mind over matter."

Dr. Laverne Johnson, a Stanford alumnus, had read about this experiment and had volunteered his laboratory at the San Diego Naval Hospital. There, at 6:12 a.m., precisely 264 hours and 12 minutes after his alarm clock had awakened him eleven days earlier, Randy Gardner went to sleep. I must admit that I didn't have the faintest idea about how long he would stay asleep, and I certainly didn't know what to tell the hordes of reporters who buzzed about demanding predictions. Randy slept for only fourteen hours and forty minutes, and when he awoke he was essentially recovered. He was actually up and out at 10 p.m. and stayed awake without difficulty until the next night, which was about twenty-four hours. His second sleep after the long vigil was eight hours and seemed quite normal. He has since been followed by Dr. Johnson, for whom he worked in the ensuing years, and appears to be completely healthy and unaffected by the experience—except for whatever effect being a transient national celebrity may have had on his psyche. Except for a few illusions—one or two minor hallucinatory experiences—Randy demonstrated no psychotic behavior during the entire vigil, no paranoid behavior, no serious emotional change.

The crucial factor in surmounting the effects of prolonged sleep loss is probably physical fitness. There is almost no degree of sleepiness that cannot be overcome if the subject engages in vigorous exercise. As the vigil wears on, almost continuous muscular activity is necessary to forestall overwhelming sleepiness. Many individuals simply would not be able to maintain this amount of activity, and would therefore appear to succumb to the debilitating effects of sleep loss. Although the elderly are said to require less sleep, deprivation studies have not been done in such individuals for obvious reasons. However, some years ago, Wilse Webb of the University of Florida showed that elderly rats could not tolerate prolonged wakefulness.

At any rate, if the subject is highly motivated and in top physical condition, as was Randy Gardner, we have begun to suspect that the vigil could go on indefinitely. Does this prove that sleep is not really necessary? Unfortunately, researchers have demonstrated the existence of momentary lapses called "microsleeps" during these prolonged vigils. Continuous observations of telemetered physiological data will be needed to be absolutely sure in future studies that the microsleeps throughout the day do not add up to substantial amounts of somnolence.

The occurrence of transient mental derangement in some subjects undergoing prolonged sleep loss is not easy to explain. We will return to this subject in Chapter Five, but for the moment we may offer the comment that some individuals are predisposed to this kind of breakdown in the face of almost any stressful experience.

Mechanism of Sleep

Perhaps the most intriguing event of the night is the passage from the last moment of wakefulness to the first moment of sleep. We think of going to sleep as a gradual process—a slow descent into oblivion through a kaleidoscopic reverie of half-formed images and undefined sensations. Yet, the onset of sleep is not "gradual." It happens in an instant. One second the organism is aware—the next second it is not. Awareness stops abruptly, as if 10 billion furiously communicating brain cells were suddenly placed on "stand-by" status.

Nearly all discussions of the mechanism of sleep emphasize the central nervous system and assume that the body is guided and regulated by the brain and spinal cord. The brain itself must be controlled in order to regulate sleep-waking behavior. The crucial regulating centers are thought to be in the brain stem, a small area about the size of one's little finger located at the base of the brain. This is the area that connects the spinal cord with the rest of the brain, controls the movements of the eyes, and receives the input of all the cranial nerves. (See Figure 1. Figures begin on page 106.)

Several hypotheses have been set forth to explain how man passes from wakefulness to sleep and back to wakefulness. One consideration concerns some rather old notions about the natural state of the brain. Some viewed it as active and felt that the state of activity had to be interrupted periodically in the interest of restoration and recovery. This was primarily the teaching of Ivan Pavlov, the noted Russian neurophysiologist who founded the conditioned response school of psychology.

Another school would prefer to view the natural state of the brain as resting—the brain must be urged into activity by some agency or need to respond. Kleitman was one of the foremost proponents of this view. He felt that the problem was not to explain sleep but to explain wakefulness. It seemed obvious to him, as a result of his sleep deprivation studies, that muscular activity and sensory bombardment are necessary to maintain wakefulness. By retiring to a quiet room, switching off the lights, removing constricting clothing, lying down, and closing our eyes, we bring about a drastic reduction of sensory stimulation. In the absence of this sensory bombardment, the activity of the nervous system passively falls below some critical level and sleep naturally ensues.

Further development of this notion came with the discovery that a crucial structure was interposed between the higher centers of the brain and the sensory input. This structure was the reticular formation of the brain stem, which was found to receive collaterals from the sensory pathways together with fibers from the higher brain centers. By adding its own intrinsic activity, this reticular formation, or waking center, might control changes in waking or sleeping behavior with a great deal of independence from outside stimuli. Thus, we hypothesize that the reticular formation contains a system whose activity induces and maintains wakefulness and whose inactivity leads to sleep.

The notion of a sleep-inducing system was further enhanced by the contribution of Michel Jouvet, professor of experimental medicine at the University of Lyon, whose work hinges on the hypothetical role of serotonin and serotonergic neurons in the brain stem. (Readers—those of you who have a passion for neurochemistry will someday have to regroup with me for a private discussion as it would surely drive the rest of our literary public into folding this book. We will, however, discuss the exciting implications of this research in Chapter Six.)

My own philosophy involves a pacemaker theory of sleep. As we have noted, some scientists hold that the brain requires a system, probably located in the brain stem, to put it to sleep; I believe that, if the crucial areas of brain stem were destroyed, other areas could take on this function. An analogy may be made with the heart and its pacemaker system. The sinus node is the pacemaker of the heart, but if it is destroyed the atrium takes over. If the atrium is destroyed, the ventricle takes over. The pace may be a little slower, but the inherent rhythmicity is present. Because circadian rhythms (daily, cyclical fluctuations) are presumed to be innately present in every living cell, there is no reason why such a notion would not be viable. We could assume that every cell in the brain has an independent capacity to be "awake" or "asleep."

Function of Sleep

"Common sense" tells us that sleep results from fatigue and fatigue results from activity, but this assumed relationship between sleep and physical exertion has been undermined by observing people who are in bed twenty-four hours a day. It appears that they do not sleep substantially less than the rest of us. The objection has been raised that bed rest itself is somehow fatiguing.

Several imaginative investigators have attempted to learn something about the function of sleep by studying persons placed in environments where fatigue was virtually eliminated. One example is a study made in the late 1950s by a trio of scientists connected with the Air Force. They observed sleep in a "hydrodynamic environment." The subject remained seated on a reclining chair in a large pool of water heated to body temperature. With his limbs totally supported, he floated for twenty-three hours out of twenty-four hours (with one hour out for routine toilet activities). The subject reduced his sleep time from about seven hours a day to a little more than three hours a day. During the day the subject engaged in a number of psychomotor tasks, and his performance remained unimpaired. He showed no tiredness as a result of this reduction in sleep time. Unfortunately, this result was never reproduced in another laboratory. However, the ultimate experiment of this kind has since been performed. This was the absolute weightlessness experienced by the Apollo astronauts on their various trips to the moon and back. Although the complete details are not available, my friends in the National Aeronautics and Space Administration (NASA) have led me to believe that the reduction in sleep time was unremarkable. Thus, while it is true that muscular fatigue will be ameliorated while the body is "at rest" during the night, it seems clear that the reversal of fatigue is not the specific function of sleep or the sole reason for its existence.

We have many times alluded to the important role of activity and stimulation in maintaining wakefulness during prolonged vigils. Does this mean that a subject's sleep time would be greatly increased if we could remove all sensory stimulation from his environment? (While this may at first seem to contradict the "fatigue theory," which might predict the opposite, the current question deals with visual and auditory rather than muscular activity.)

Rather interesting results on the removal of sensory stimulation were obtained by Dr. Royce Royal and his colleagues at the United States Naval Hospital at Bethesda, Maryland. In their study, volunteers were placed in soundproof rooms which were totally silent and completely dark—one volunteer to a room. They wore gloves to reduce tactile sensations. A chemical toilet and a food locker, which the subjects could operate, enabled them to remain in this situation twenty-four hours a day. Once or twice a day the experimenters communicated with the subjects for the purpose of psychomotor testing, and there was continuous monitoring so that the subjects could come out if they wished.

Under these circumstances, the subjects had little to do but sleep. On the first day they slept a mean of between twelve and fourteen hours. (The subjects, young Navy recruits, may have been somewhat tired when they entered the isolation chamber.) But in the course of seven days the total sleep time gradually decreased until the mean on the last two days was six hours or less per day. The supposition is that sensory isolation ultimately favors wakefulness; and this may suggest inferentially that wakefulness is the basic state of the brain.

In spite of many heroic efforts, sleep researchers have failed, to date, to define the function of sleep. This fact elicited some interesting commentary from my close friend Allan Rechtschaffen, sleep researcher, professor of psychology (and incidentally bon vivant) from the University of Chicago:

> Perhaps sleep does not have a function. Perhaps, as some of my own students have argued with me, we should accept our failure to isolate a specific function for sleep as evidence for nonexistence of such a function, but it is hard to believe that we spend almost one-third of our lives in a behavioral state that has no function at all. It is hard to believe that the unrelenting pressure for sleep after we have been deprived of it is not the work of a sensitive need system that reacts quickly and powerfully to deprivation.
>
> If sleep does not serve an absolutely vital function, then it is the biggest mistake the evolutionary process ever made. Sleep precludes hunting for and consuming food. It is incompatible with procreation. It produces vulnerability to attack from enemies. Sleep interferes with every voluntary adaptive motor act in the repertoire of coping mechanisms. How could natural selection with its irrevocable logic have "permitted" the animal kingdom to pay the price of sleep for no good reason? In fact, the behavior of sleep is so apparently maladaptive that one can only wonder why some other condition did not evolve to satisfy whatever need it is that sleep satisfies. Is sleep only a vestigial remnant which has outlived its functional usefulness? Probably not. How could sleep have remained virtually unchanged as a monstrously useless, maladaptive vestige throughout the whole of mammalian evolution while selection has, during the same period of time, been able to achieve all kinds of delicate, finely tuned adjustments in the shape of fingers and toes? (From "The Control of Sleep" by Allan Rechtschaffen, in *Human Behavior and its Control*, William A. Hunt, ed., Cambridge, Mass: Schenkman Publishing Co., 1971.)

Circadian Rhythms

Even though we do not at present understand the vital function of sleep, it is clear that it is an integral part of the rhythm of our daily lives. Night follows day, day follows night, and even if we do not sleep,

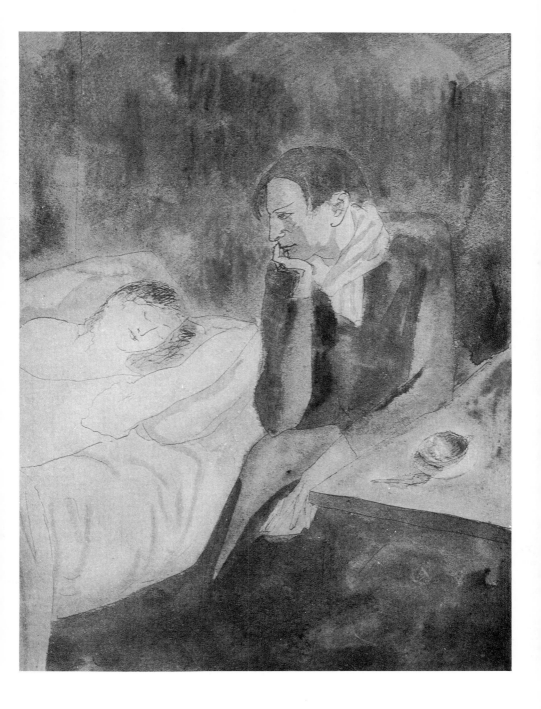

the sleep-wakefulness rhythm continues in the form of a profound fluctuation in sleepiness and alertness. (Figure 2)

Our entire world is engaged in rhythm. We observe rhythmicity in the tides, in the rising and setting of sun and moon, in the seasons of the year, and even in the stock market. The temporal organization of all animals is influenced by the endless succession of day and night as the rotation of the earth imposes its daily cycle.

Stanford Professor of Biology Colin Pittendrigh, an international figure in the study of circadian rhythms, demonstrates to class after class that all organisms, from the single cell to man, are innately oscillatory in their time course. This fact was not generally known until well into our twentieth century; yet it is one of the most basic factors carried forward in the evolution of life. (Some scientists speculate that it takes about twenty-four hours for a complete genetic read-out, when all the DNA in chromosomes forms the messenger RNA.) In man, more than one hundred functions and structural elements can be named which oscillate between maximal and minimal values once a day. They range from the well-known rhythm in deep body temperature to rhythms in mood and mental performance. In addition, the peaks and troughs of the individual oscillators may occur at unique times that are different from one another.

Body temperature, for example, peaks during the middle of the day and falls to its lowest point during the early-morning hours. Anyone required to stay up all night experiences this temperature change by feeling chilly around 4 a.m., even in a well heated room. Performance tests completed in the middle of the night show much poorer scores than those taken at midday. This performance decrement is not due to sleep loss only; higher scores are obtained at noon on a day following twenty-four hours of sleep deprivation than at 4 a.m. following only six hours of sleep loss. We are all more or less inept during the nighttime hours.

It has been experimentally demonstrated that these twenty-four hour cycles are based on endogenous, self-sustained oscillations. Under constant conditions, as for example in an underground bunker where temperature and humidity are maintained at a single value, the organism *continues* to oscillate, but at its own natural or innate frequency. The period of such a "free running" rhythm usually deviates slightly from that of the earth's rotation; i.e., from twenty-four hours. The word "circadian"—*circa*, around; *dies*, day—was coined by Dr. Franz Halberg to cover these rhythms which under natural conditions are entrained to twenty-four hours by the synchronizing effects of the environment. Professor Jurgen Aschoff at the Max Planck Institute in Munich has shown that man has an innate oscillatory frequency of about twenty-five hours in a constant environment. He has also shown that these rhythms in man can be entrained to periods one or two hours shorter or longer than the natural frequency, but that synchronized oscillation cannot be achieved at periodicities substantially different from twenty-five hours, with one exception. About one person in twenty can achieve a normal physiological cycle with a periodicity of forty-eight hours!

The sleepiness we feel after several nights—or even one night—of restricted or lost sleep may be due not to the lack of sufficient sleep but to a phase shift of our circadian rhythms. The now-familiar "jet-lag syndrome" is an example of a phase shift. If one flies from San Francisco to New York and then goes to bed at 11 p.m. E.S.T., he may have trouble falling asleep because his body is still operating on Pacific Time. Even though he obtains eight hours' sleep that night, he may find it difficult to awaken at seven o'clock (E.S.T.) because it is only 4 a.m. to his body. If the jet traveler stays in New York for several days, however, his body will adjust to the new schedule. When he jets back to San Francisco, his body functions are now three hours ahead of the West Coast clock schedule, and again he needs a few days to adjust. A phase shift does not necessarily involve a loss of sleep; it means that "body time" is out-of-phase with "clock time."

It is no great imaginative leap to suggest that feeling sleepy might have as much to do with the phase of the circadian rhythm as with sleep loss. In addition, such things as phase shift and internal desynchronization (when two or more physiological oscillators in a single individual begin to fluctuate with totally different periodicities) have great relevance for sleep problems such as insomnia and hypersomnia.

It has been said that sleep "is to prevent us from wandering around in the dark and bumping into things." Perhaps it is true that our primitive ancestor used sleep as a place to hide from the terrors of the night. It is also true that he slept during the hours when he was least efficient, during the depressed phase of his circadian rhythm.

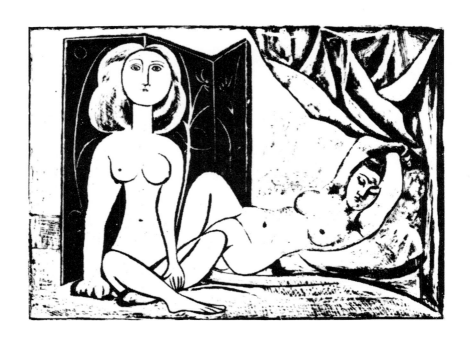

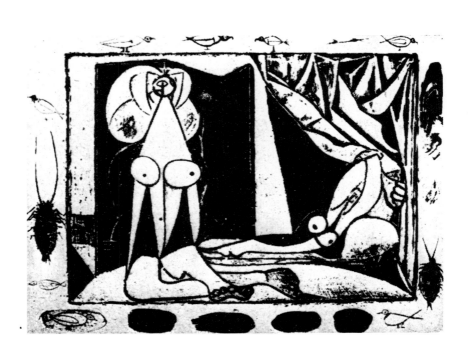

CHAPTER TWO

TWO KINDS OF SLEEP

EARLY SLEEP RESEARCHERS FACED an insurmountable problem: it was almost impossible to study sleep without awakening the sleeper! They tried taking the subject's blood pressure or "gently" prying open his eyelids to see if his pupils were dilated. Obviously it's impossible to study sleep in a subject who has just been rudely awakened. This problem remained unsolved until brain wave techniques became available in the 1930s.

It must have been difficult in those early days to find individuals who were willing to be poked and prodded all night long in the interest of medical science. Many of the early researchers tried to experiment on themselves—but of course it isn't easy to study sleep while sleeping.

The history of sleep research is peopled with intrepid adventurers who were willing to study—or slumber—under unusual conditions and in exotic locales in order to learn more about sleep. Some of these studies were designed to learn the effects of sleep-waking cycles that were not based upon the twenty-four-hour day. Could man adjust to a twenty-eight-hour day, for example, with nineteen hours for waking activity and nine hours for sleep?

Nathaniel Kleitman and B. H. Richardson put themselves on this schedule in the murky interior of Mammoth Cave in Central Kentucky. Cut off from the outside world, except for food deliveries, they regularly sampled their body temperatures and carefully evaluated their sleep. Their sleep was rated poorest when the innate rhythm of body temperature was not synchronous with the artificial sleep-wakefulness schedule. In the early part of this century, other investigators conducted similar studies in the darkness of Greenland's winter and in the continual daylight of summer in Tromsö, Norway.

Modern-day sleep research has also been conducted in some very out-of-the-way places. Telemetry has allowed the monitoring of sleep in space, on the moon, on mountain tops, and in submarines. Special laboratories have been constructed in underground bunkers. By maintaining sleep laboratories on two continents, investigators are now studying the effects of jet travel on sleep.

Since contemporary sleep laboratories throughout the world are quite similar to one another, let us use the Stanford University Sleep Laboratory as an example of such facilities. The Stanford lab consists of six bedrooms, all connected to a larger room in which monitoring devices are located. Carpeted and tastefully decorated, the bedrooms are made to seem "like home." In addition, they are soundproof, temperature-controlled, and pitch black when the lights are turned off.

Although the rooms are attractive and the scientific equipment is almost entirely hidden, it is still hard to find volunteers willing to sleep in them. People are reluctant to spend a night or a series of nights away from their homes and their families, to sleep in a strange bed in an unfamiliar setting, and to be observed while they sleep. Consequently, the majority of subjects who volunteer for sleep studies are college students to whom the promise of five or ten dollars a night ("Just to sleep?") is a great incentive.

How Sleep is Measured

In order to identify and classify sleep, it is necessary to record the electrical activity of three systems: the brain, the eyes, and the muscles. These systems are monitored simultaneously by an instrument called the polygraph, which allows measurements to be made continuously throughout the night without disturbing the sleeping subject. Tiny electrodes attached to the scalp and face of the subject convey signals to the polygraph where they are recorded on moving chart paper by pens that move up and down automatically in response to changes in electrical potentials. (Figure 3)

The up-and-down movement of the pens and the lateral movement of the paper produces a pattern of waves. These waves are meaningless scribbles to the uninformed observer, but if they are recorded in a standard and conventional manner, a night of sleep can be interpreted accurately by any knowledgeable researcher. In somewhat the manner of the experienced surfer watching ocean waves, the sleep researcher looks for changes in form and frequency of brain waves.

The record of brain activity is called *electroencephalogram* or EEG. The polygraph records the voltage fluctuations between two points on the scalp or, in the case of animals, within the brain itself. The record of eye movements is called an *electrooculogram* or EOG. The eyes are like tiny batteries with a difference of electrical potential between the cornea and the retina. Changes of the electrical field are recorded as transorbital potential differences whenever the eyes move. The record of muscle activity is called an *electromyogram* (EMG). It shows the electrical potentials generated in the muscle fibers.

In routine studies of nocturnal sleep, the subject arrives at the laboratory about an hour before his usual bedtime. He prepares for bed by going through the same bedtime ritual he is accustomed to at home, while the experimenter checks the equipment. When the subject is ready for bed, the experimenter begins the routine application of electrodes. All of this must be completed, and fail-safe, before the subject goes to sleep so it will not be necessary to make adjustments in the middle of the night and therefore disturb the normal sleep pattern. In certain subjects or patients, these recordings are continued around-the-clock for many days, and the subject essentially lives in the laboratory.

The first step in the electrode attachment is a thorough cleansing of the skin or scalp with acetone or alcohol at points where the electrodes are to be placed. Scalp electrodes are attached by means of a cotton or gauze pad soaked in collodion and quick-dried with a flow of compressed air. Surgical tape is used to attach the electrodes to facial regions. When all the electrodes are in place, the wires are brought together into a bundle and anchored to the scalp in a kind of "pony tail," which the subject carries with him when he retires to bed. The experimenter plugs each of the wires into a numbered panel on the headboard, which is connected by cable to a similar panel on the polygraph. By using corresponding numbers, the experimenter can "tune in" the appropriate channels on the polygraph as if it were a television set.

After a final equipment check, the experimenter wishes the subject a good night's sleep, turns off the light, and closes the door as he departs. By the time the subject awakens in the morning—to be greeted by a sleepy-eyed experimenter—nearly one thousand feet of chart paper or magnetic tape will have been traced with a record of brain waves, eye movements, and muscle activity. (Figure 4) Although the subject may experience minor discomfort from the electrodes taped to his face, there is no pain involved in sleep recording, and at no time is any current flowing from the polygraph to the subject.

In addition to studying human sleep, we study the sleep effects of various drugs and surgical procedures in cats, rats, hampsters, mice, and monkeys. Although it is often necessary to implant electrodes into the brains of cats, the procedures we use are not painful to the cats. When the study is completed, we are usually able to remove the electrodes and to "rehabilitate" the animals as house pets. Unfortunately, we sometimes experience considerable difficulty finding homes for our "rehabilitated veterans." When this happens, some member of the laboratory staff (occasionally this author) adds one more cat to the household menagerie.

There are people who simply cannot condone any kind of experimentation performed upon animals. I receive a great deal of hate mail, including threats upon my life, from some of these animal lovers. One letter writer warned that he will be stalking me with a high-powered rifle! We believe that some use of animals is necessary to advance our knowledge of normal and pathological states, but I can readily assure the reader that we have never caused an animal to suffer.

The Discovery of REM Sleep

Every day every human being—every mammal, in fact—experiences two kinds of sleep that alternate rhythmically throughout the entire sleep period. These two kinds of sleep are as different from each other as sleep is from wakefulness. If there is a cat or a dog in your household, chances are you have observed the two states of sleep many times. At one moment the sleeping animal seems to be lifeless except for its regular breathing. Then the breathing becomes irregular, paws and whiskers begin to twitch, lips and tongue begin to move—and someone says, "Oh, look at Rover! He's *dreaming*!"

The discovery of the two kinds of sleep occurred almost accidentally at the University of Chicago. In 1952 Dr. Kleitman became interested in the slow rolling eye movements that accompany sleep onset and decided to look for these eye movements throughout the night to determine whether they were related to the depth or quality of sleep. Kleitman gave the assignment of watching eye movements to one of his graduate students in the department of physiology, Eugene Aserinsky.

The young student soon noticed an entirely new kind of eye movement. At certain times during the night, the eyes began to dart about furiously beneath the closed lids. These unexpected episodes were startlingly different from the familiar slow, pendular movements that were the original object of the study.

Over the years, many people have asked me, "How can you see the eye moving when the lids are closed?" As a matter of fact, it is very easy to see eye movements when the eyes are closed. Have someone do it and see for yourself. However, Aserinsky was using the polygraph to monitor the subject, and the eye movements were actually discovered on the chart paper. It was not until he directly observed these movements in sleeping subjects that he could believe the spectacular inked-out deviations. It would be difficult today to understand how skeptical we were. These eye movements, which had all the attributes of waking eye movements, had absolutely no business appearing in sleep. In those days, sleep was conceived of as a state of neural depression or inhibition—quiescence, rest. It was definitely not a condition in which the brain could be generating highly coordinated eye movements that were, in many instances, faster and sharper than the subject could execute while awake.

I have always felt that this was *the* breakthrough—the discovery that changed the course of sleep research from a relatively pedestrian inquiry into an intensely exciting endeavor pursued with great determination in laboratories and clinics all over the world. And there is nothing more exciting to a researcher than findings that are totally different from what he had expected.

Of course, the change in all our concepts of sleep didn't occur overnight. Having joined the research effort at this point as a sophomore medical student under Kleitman, I began to record the electroencephalograph and other physiological variables, along with eye movement activity. Since I didn't know what to expect, I kept my eyes glued to the moving chart paper all night long. After many nights, certain definite relationships were discernible in the enormous amounts of data. Rapid eye movements were always accompanied by very distinctive brain wave patterns, a change in breathing, and other striking departures from the normal, quiet sleep pattern. In addition, what we now call the basic ninety-minute sleep pattern began to emerge from the night-to-night variability.

As more and more physiological changes were discovered and described, we realized that sleep was *not* a quiet resting state that continued without variance as long as the subject was fortunate enough to remain asleep. No. For the first time we realized what has probably been true of man's sleep since he crawled out of the primordial slime. Man has *two* kinds of sleep. His nocturnal solitude contains two entirely different phenomena.

REM and NREM Sleep

I coined the term "REM" (for rapid-eye-movement) sleep to define the phenomenon my colleagues and I had observed. The other kind of sleep eventually acquired the name "NREM" (pronounced non-REM) sleep.

Most of the changes typically associated with falling asleep are the consequence of reclining and relaxing. Cardiac and respiratory rates will decrease, body temperature will fall, blood pressure will decline, and metabolic activity will drop. If we continue to lie still and relax, we may fall asleep without the occurrence of any further changes.

The NREM state is often called "quiet sleep" because of the slow, regular breathing, the general absence of body movement, and the slow, regular brain activity shown in the EEG. It is important to remember that the body is not paralyzed during NREM sleep; it *can* move, but it *does not* move because the brain doesn't order it to move. The sleeper has lost contact with his environment. There is a shut-down of perception because the five senses are no longer gathering information and communicating stimuli to the brain. When gross body movements (such as rolling over) occur during NREM, the EEG suggests a transient intrusion of wakefulness—yet the individual may not be responsive at the time, nor recall having moved if subsequently awakened. In one respect the term "quiet sleep" is a misnomer: it is during NREM sleep that snoring occurs.

REM sleep, which has been called "active sleep," is an entirely different state of existence. At the onset of REM sleep, the sleeper's body is still immobile, but we can see small, convulsive twitches of his face and fingertips. His snoring ceases, and his breathing becomes irregular —very fast, then slow—he may even appear to stop breathing for several seconds. Under the eyelids the corneal bulges of his eyes dart around, back and forth. If we gently pull back the eyelids, the subject seems to be actually looking at something. Cerebral blood flow and brain temperature soar to new heights, but the large muscles of the body are completely paralyzed; arms, legs, and trunk cannot move. Throbbing penile erections occur in adult—and newborn—males.

There is some speculation that REM sleep is not really sleep at all, but a state in which the subject is awake, but paralyzed and hallucinating. (Some evidence for this point of view exists in narcolepsy, an illness we'll discuss in Chapter Five.)

All of the short-lived events or bursts of activity that occur *within* the periods of REM sleep—individual eye movements, muscle twitches, and so forth—are collectively called phasic activity. This includes short-lived contractions of the middle ear muscles that occur in sleep only during the REM state. These contractions are identical with middle ear muscle activity seen in wakefulness as a response to various intensities and pitches of sound. In the cat, researchers may have located the primary phasic activity—the one that triggers all the others. It is an electrical event called the PGO spike. The acronym stands for pons, geniculate bodies, and occipital cortex—areas of the brain where the electrical spike is recorded during REM periods. Although it has so far been impossible in humans to get recordings from the depth of the brain, Rechtschaffen has discovered, in both humans and cats, a REM phasic activity that may be closely associated with PGO spikes. This event, known as phasic integrated potential (PIP), is a sharp shift in electrical potential recorded from the muscles surrounding the eyes.

All of these discoveries are helping to bring the mystery of REM sleep—and maybe even the fantasy of dreams—out of the shadowy dusk of speculation and into the clear bright light of observable phenomena. Sometimes it seems a shame, to anyone who believes that mystery and fantasy enrich our lives. Nonetheless, a researcher is obliged to state the facts—to describe phenomena in terms of what we know. Speaking in such a strict manner with regard to REM sleep, I can only say: "It's there. It looks the way I've described it." We just don't know yet, despite twenty years of intensive research, *why* it's there. In many ways, REM periods resemble epileptic seizures. Perhaps they are equally useful.

Course of Events During the Night

Frequently associated with the reverie of sleep onset is a feeling of floating or falling, which often terminates abruptly in a jerk returning us to wakefulness. Such starts, called myoclonias, generally occur only during the first five minutes of sleep and are a normal occurrence, seemingly more prevalent in "nervous" people. On some occasions the myoclonia may be an arousal response to a very weak, insignificant external stimulus.

Even with an EEG reading it is impossible to pinpoint the exact instant of sleep onset. The essential difference between wakefulness and sleep is the loss of awareness. Sleep onset occurs at the exact instant when a meaningful stimulus fails to elicit its accustomed response. (This does not mean that no response whatsoever can be obtained. A stimulus of sufficient magnitude or significance, such as a loud noise or the soft calling of one's name, elicits a very definite response: arousal.)

A dramatic illustration of the nature of sleep onset has been obtained in the laboratory through the use of visual stimuli. A sleepy subject lies in bed with his eyes taped open (which can be achieved, believe it or not, with relatively little discomfort). A very bright strobe light is placed about six inches in front of his face and is flashed into his eyes at the rate of about once every second or two. A microswitch is taped to his finger, which he is instructed to press every time he sees a flash. A simple task. How can he possibly avoid seeing the flash? The subject will press and press. Suddenly he stops. If we immediately ask why, he will be surprised. The light exploded right into his widely open eyes, yet he was totally unaware. In one second, he was awake, seeing, hearing, responding—in the very next second, he was functionally blind and asleep.

At the moment when visual perception ceases, the eyes begin to drift slowly from side to side either synchronously or asynchronously. This slow rolling of the eyes is one of the most reliable signs of the onset of sleep. The first sleep of the night is always NREM sleep, which must progress through its various stages before the first REM period occurs. Along with the slowly rolling eye movements, we see a gradual transition in the pattern of EEG waves from the characteristic rhythm of wakefulness to the NREM Stage 1 configuration.

What follows is a progressive descent from Stage 1 into other stages of NREM sleep. The term "descent" is meant to imply a progression along the depth-of-sleep continuum as sleep becomes deeper and deeper, the sleeper becomes more remote from the environment, and increasingly more potent stimuli are necessary to cause arousal.

Each new stage is announced by its own characteristic pattern in the EEG. After only a few minutes of Stage 1, the onset of Stage 2 is established by the appearance of spindling and K complexes. Several minutes later the slow delta waves of Stage 3 become apparent. After about ten minutes of this stage, the delta activity becomes more and more predominant and signals the presence of Stage 4. At this point it is extremely difficult to awaken the sleeper. A child in this stage of sleep is virtually unreachable and may take several minutes to return to full awareness if he can be aroused at all. It is during this period that sleep-talking, sleepwalking, night terrors, and bed-wetting are initiated in young children.

In Stage 4, thirty or forty minutes following sleep onset, a series of body movements heralds the start of a re-ascent through the stages of NREM sleep. Approximately seventy or eighty minutes from the onset of sleep the Stage 1 EEG pattern occurs again. But now there are sawtooth waves in the EEG, rapid eye movements in the EOG, a suppression of activity in the EMG, and a host of other physiological changes. The first REM period has begun. It will last about ten minutes.

Throughout the night this cyclic variation between NREM and REM sleep continues. The NREM-REM cycle varies from seventy to 110 minutes but averages around ninety minutes. In the early part of the night, sleep is dominated by the NREM state, particularly Stages 3 and 4, but as the night wears on, REM sleep periods become progressively longer, sometimes as long as sixty minutes, and Stage 2 represents the only NREM interruption.

An adult who sleeps seven and one-half hours each night generally spends one and one-half to two hours in REM sleep. Since people who are awakened during REM periods usually recall a dream, it can be said that we dream roughly every ninety minutes all night long. After offering us several short episodes early in the night, the brain may produce an hour-long "feature film."

Phylogeny (Who Has REM Sleep?)

We are often asked, "Do plants sleep?" We can't really answer this except to say that sleep and wakefulness are primarily manifestations of the brain, and since plants do not have brains, these terms do not apply. Even in amphibians, who are considerably higher on the phylo-

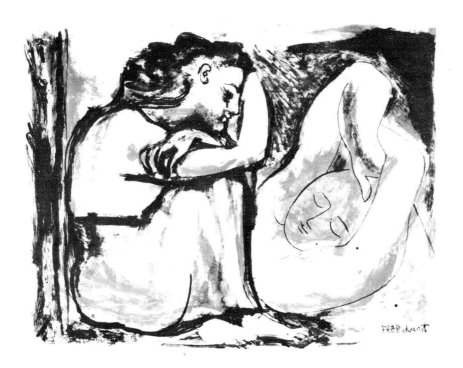

genetic scale than insects and fish, we cannot clearly define sleep and waking states (as opposed to mere quiescence and activity). For example, when the frog is active, it shows sleep-like brain waves, and when it appears to be asleep, its brain waves look awake. Most reptiles appear to have NREM sleep as we know it, but *do not* show any REM sleep at all. Birds have very well developed NREM sleep, and show occasional, very brief (about one second) episodes of what appears to be an evolutionary precursor of the REM period. Full-blown REM periods exist only in mammalian sleep. Interestingly enough, all mammals appear to have substantial amounts of REM sleep, and whatever differences may exist between individual species do not follow any readily apparent rule. According to Dr. Frederick Snyder, the oppossum —one of the most primitive mammals, often called a "living fossil"— has as much as or more REM sleep than man. A few of the many species whose sleep has been carefully studied are elephant, chimpanzee, whale, shrew, pig, sheep, monkey, rat, mouse, cat, bat, dog, donkey, guinea pig, and human. Some non-mammals that have been observed by sleep researchers are frog, alligator, lizard, various fish, pigeon, chicken, eagle, and snake.

Ontogeny

One of the most remarkable aspects of REM sleep is the very large amount that is present in most mammals immediately after birth. In the newborn human baby who sleeps an average of sixteen to eighteen hours per day, at least 50 percent of all this sleep (eight to nine hours!) is occupied by REM periods. People invariably ask, "What can they be dreaming about in all that time?" The occurrence of so much REM sleep in newborn infants will raise some difficult questions about the relationship of REM sleep, rapid eye movements, and dreaming (see next chapter).

In premature infants of thirty-two to thirty-six weeks gestation, the percent of REM sleep is even higher, around 75 percent of the total amount of sleep. This finding suggests that there is a phase in the early intrauterine life of the child when REM sleep is the all-encompassing mode of existence.

After birth, the amount of REM sleep declines gradually and reaches the level of about 25 percent of the total sleep time at around five years of age. From age five to adulthood, Stage 4 predominates.

In some animals, the predominance of REM sleep in early life is even more spectacular. For example, in the newborn kitten, REM sleep is the *only* sleep. This is also true of the newborn puppy, rat, and hamster.

On the other hand, the newborn guinea pig has very little REM sleep.

Because of the extraordinary amount of REM sleep in infants and our difficulty in demonstrating the purpose of REM sleep in adults, we cannot help wondering if the real function of REM sleep is fulfilled early in life. Perhaps REM sleep is necessary for the normal pre- and post-natal maturation of the brain. This fits with the guinea pig data because this animal is "mature" at birth.

A REM Sleep Theory

The pessimistic opinion that there may be no useful function to REM sleep makes a pretty poor springboard for scientific inquiry. You must posit *something* before you begin any realistic investigation. The puzzle of REM sleep has prompted numerous theories, and one of the most ingenious experiments I know of was carried out by a group of freshman students at Stanford. They were enrolled in our Sleep and Dream course and their names (so they may claim credit for their lovely piece of work, if they wish) are Sally Carpenter, Joy Kelley, Evan Laughlin, Robert Lenz, Kathy Sidoric, and Joy Simmons.

They proceeded on this basis: One of the general advantages of sleep is calorie conservation. Simply put, the more an animal sleeps, the less it must eat. One of the things we do know about sleep is that the duration of NREM sleep, which accomplishes body rest and quiescence, is limited. The brain can only operate in this quiet mode for one or two hours, then it must switch to an active mode for at least ten or twenty minutes before the quiet can be re-established. The students theorized that REM periods might be a special state enabling the brain to be active while maintaining quiescence and calorie conservation through a blockade of muscle function. Thus, the regular alternation of NREM and REM periods enables the average person to sleep all night, instead of waking at the end of each NREM period in response to the brain's need to return to an active mode. If instead of sleeping through the night one were to awaken for regular "active" intervals, the need for REM sleep might disappear, or drastically diminish. The students designed an experiment to test this hypothesis. Choosing the basic ninety-minute sleep cycle (remember on the average there is one NREM period in every ninety minutes of normal sleep), they designed a ninety-minute day in which there would be sixty minutes of wakefulness followed by thirty minutes of sleep. If the wakefulness periods performed the activating function which the students had posited to REM sleep, someone living on such a schedule would bypass the need for REM sleep. *Would it work?*

Joy Kelley, a healthy eighteen-year-old, volunteered to live on the ninety-minute day for as long as six consecutive real days. During the course of the study, she lived in the Stanford University Sleep Laboratory, partly isolated from environmental influences. Every ninety minutes she went to bed for a thirty-minute sleep, after which she was awake for an hour. Her fellow students monitored her sleep polygraphically and, during the waking periods, tested her blood pressure, pulse, mood, and motor balance. Joy rated each successive fifteen-minute period of wakefulness on the Stanford Sleepiness Scale, which is divided into seven degrees of sleepiness ranging from "wide awake" to "almost in reverie," and completed questionnaires relating to the overall quality of each sleeping and waking interval. The student monitors maintained a log book in which they commented upon Joy's general level of functioning during each "day."

The study began with the first thirty-minute sleep period when Joy went to bed at 2:10 a.m. after a normal full day of wakefulness. The last thirty-minute sleep period started at 5:30 p.m. on the sixth day, after which she spent approximately seven hours awake (because of an examination). Joy then returned to her regular circadian schedule of sleep and wakefulness with all-night sleep recordings made on two consecutive "recovery" nights. Two months after the experiment she returned to the sleep laboratory and was recorded for two "baseline" nights. (It is important to note that the experimental manipulation was not terminated because of any discomfort, either physical or mental, on the part of the subject, but was dictated by prior commitments and academic requirements.)

The results of the ninety-minute-day study show that Joy was able to shift to the new sleep-waking schedule with remarkable ease. She failed to sleep on only one of the ninety-one "nights" while on the regime. In spite of the relative inefficiency of breaking her sleep allotment into sixteen separate periods, she obtained more than five hours of total sleep time during each of the twenty-four-hour periods except the first one, in which she had four hours and nineteen minutes of sleep, including thirty minutes of Stage 4 sleep but no REM sleep at all. Stage 4 quickly attained higher levels and averaged 11.1 percent thereafter. REM periods were recorded on fifteen of the ninety-one "nights" and appeared after only a few minutes of NREM sleep or, on several occasions, at sleep onset! By the last two twenty-four-hour periods, REM sleep had attained levels of 20.1 percent and 18.3 percent of total sleep time. These levels were slightly above the baseline.

It has been suggested that the alternation of REM and NREM sleep is the nighttime phase of a basic rest-activity cycle (BRAC) that exists in masked form throughout the day. Presumably, we become more active at ninety-minute intervals both day and night. If such a ninety-minute BRAC is present, the subject of an experiment like ours would presumably slip easily into a ninety-minute sleep-wakefulness cycle. The remarkable ease with which Joy adjusted to this schedule—her ability to sleep on all but one of the "nights" and her general feeling of being alert on most of the "days"—may represent a confirmation of the BRAC theory. It should be noted, however, that only *one* subject was studied, and that Joy may have been unique in her ability to adjust to the schedule.

Although Joy readily adapted to the schedule, a clear-cut twenty-four hour circadian rhythm persisted throughout the experimental period. This effect was most pronounced in the timing of the sleep onset REM periods, which occurred during exactly the same clock time period in each successive twenty-four hours. Stages 3 and 4 showed a similar tendency, although the pattern was not as well established. The persistence of an overall circadian variation was clearly evident from the fact that more sleep occurred during "nights" falling between 2 a.m. and 2 p.m. than between 2 p.m. and 2 a.m.

The results of the students' experiment are really quite extraordinary. The theory that REM sleep exists to perform a sleep consolidation function was certainly not supported. Indeed, the occurrence of large amounts of REM sleep was all the more remarkable because the thirty-minute sleep periods should have entirely precluded the occurrence of REM sleep, which ordinarily does not appear in all-night sleep recordings until at least fifty to sixty minutes of NREM have elapsed. In order for Joy to have large amounts of REM sleep, she had to have REM periods at the onset of sleep. This is never seen in the nighttime sleep of normal persons, nor in daytime naps.

Does this suggest that there really is a "need" for REM sleep? A need that goes beyond merely "filling in the gaps" between NREM episodes? A need that will overcome even the most preclusive schedule? This study by Stanford students has inspired our laboratory to redouble its efforts to fathom the mysterious and elusive purpose of REM sleep.

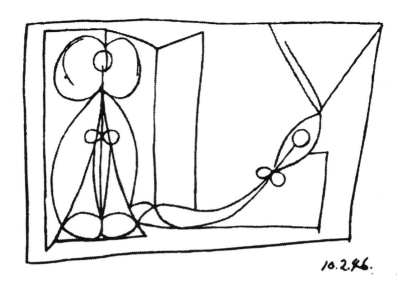

10.2.46.   I

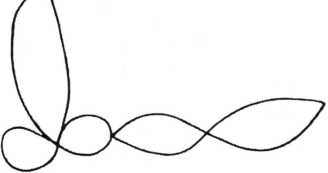

10.2.46

CHAPTER THREE

THE DREAM WORLD

FOR YEARS, SMALL GROUPS of dedicated individuals have tried to unravel the mysteries of the dream world. The superstitious dogmas of the early dream theorists gave way to the symbolism of Sigmund Freud which in turn has been succeeded by a deluge of research data filling notebooks in sleep labs all over the world. One of the most intriguing questions studied by these researchers is "What causes dreams?"

Freud wrote a marvelous review of the early dream research in his monumental work *The Interpretation of Dreams*. In Freud's day, dreams were considered the "guardians of sleep"—arising in the oblivion of sleep to protect against disrupting influences. Physiologists had defined sleep as a unitary state, but one that could vary in depth according to the amount of brain activity. When some disturbance began to impinge on sleep, there would be a partial arousal; sleep would become lighter and dreaming occurred when brain activity increased. Freud felt that a dream story, generated to incorporate the disturbing stimulus, could prevent it from fully arousing the sleeper. Thus, dreams actually protected the sleeper from inconsequential disturbances that might otherwise keep him awake half the night.

Even after REM sleep was discovered, the guardian of sleep theory persisted. Many investigators felt that the REM periods themselves must be a response to some kind of stimulus—an over-distended stomach, the need to urinate, the sudden sound of a fire siren, etc. They tested the theory—using hunger, thirst, flashing lights, dripping water, and myriad other internal and external stimuli—to see if REM sleep could be induced.

In one study done in our laboratory, we tried to see if REM sleep could be induced by bladder tension increased to a level at which it would certainly stimulate something. Our subjects drank nearly a quart of water just before going to bed, and we waited to see when they would wake up. Our results showed absolutely no relationship between the spontaneous awakening with an urgent need to urinate and the rhythmically occurring REM periods. There was occasional coincidence, but whether the bladder-filled arousal occurred in a REM period or in NREM sleep, the subjects had not dreamed of urinating.

All the studies using various stimuli showed similar results, but conclusive evidence awaited the dramatic findings in cats by Professor Michel Jouvet. Jouvet found that a very tiny electrical pulse applied to a certain portion of the cat's brain would actually produce REM sleep. But the effect disappeared if Jouvet stimulated the cat immediately following a normal REM period. In fact, Jouvet found that for about twenty minutes after each REM period, REM sleep could not be induced no matter what he tried. Thus, there appears to be a definite refractory interval after the end of REM periods during which REM sleep cannot recur.

After Jouvet demonstrated this special mechanism of REM sleep, we wanted to determine the duration of this REM sleep refractory period in humans. This was not as straightforward an undertaking as it sounds, primarily because REM periods are often quite unstable. The sleeper's REM repose may be broken by body movements and give way to intervals of wakefulness or NREM sleep. In 1962 we examined more than 1,000 REM periods and tabulated the duration of each intervening NREM interval. When we plotted the results, we obtained a dramatic U-shaped distribution. Many of the NREM intervals were very brief and many were quite long; but almost no intervals occurred in the twenty-five- to thirty-minute range. Thus, it was clear that the brief intervals of NREM sleep were essentially interruptions of single REM periods, and the long intervals were the NREM portions of the sleep cycle. In other words, once an interruption of a REM period has persisted for longer than about five minutes, there is a virtual certainty (95 to 98 percent of all instances) that the next REM interval will not take place for at least thirty minutes. The twenty-five to thirty minutes immediately following the *end* of a REM period could be labeled *completely* refractory because REM sleep apparently cannot recur during this interval. From thirty to sixty minutes after the end of the REM period could be labeled partially refractory because the probability of another REM period occurring is finite though small. As time passes, the probability increases, approaching 100 percent at around eighty minutes. Thus, the occurrence of a NREM interval longer than one hundred minutes in normal adult sleep is extremely rare. In the theory of REM sleep we considered in the previous chapter, this is what we meant by the limited duration of NREM periods.

The point of all the foregoing discussion is that *the occurrence of the REM period is determined by a physiological-biochemical process which is cyclic in nature*. Thus, REM periods and their associated dreams cannot be responses to randomly occurring internal or external disturbances.

REM Sleep and Dream Recall

For the most part, early studies of REM sleep were predicated on an interest in dreaming. Did dreaming actually occur during REM periods? Was the REM period the only time of dreaming? And, if not, how much and what kind of dream activity occurred at other times?

When Aserinsky and Kleitman first observed the rapid eye movements during sleep, it was only logical for them to infer that these ocular deviations might be related to dreaming. They tested this hypothesis by waking subjects during these periods and asking them to narrate any dream recall. The vivid recall that could be elicited in the middle of the night when a subject was awakened while his eyes were moving rapidly was nothing short of miraculous. It opened an exciting new world to the subjects whose only previous dream memories had been the vague morning-after recall. Now, instead of perhaps one fleeting glimpse into the dream world each night, the subjects could be tuned into the middle of as many as ten or twelve dreams every night.

It seemed obvious to us that REM sleep had to be the time of dreaming. But it was necessary to conduct rigorous tests of this finding—to compare arousals during REM periods with arousals during NREM sleep. Because of our expectations, the need to control bias could not have been greater. We had to be extremely careful not to lead the subjects into confirming our theory by asking questions like "What were you dreaming about?" or "You weren't dreaming, were you?" Hundreds of other tedious problems of experimental design kept our excitement in check. Nonetheless, a feeling of exhilaration prevailed in Kleitman's laboratory during the first years in which we attempted to accumulate a volume of data relating REM sleep to dreaming.

In 1957, the Kleitman lab published the fruits of these first exciting studies. We had awakened subjects 191 times during REM periods and on 152 of these awakenings, or 80 percent, we had obtained vivid dream recall! In marked contrast, during NREM periods we had awakened subjects 160 times and had obtained only eleven instances of dream recall (6.9 percent). Furthermore, in 1961 I was able to compile eight studies from the world literature that dealt with dream recall from REM and NREM awakenings. From this table (Figure 7) you can see that dream recall was obtained from 78.6 percent of the REM awakenings and almost exactly 14 percent of the NREM awakenings. After additional studies became available, we were able to report on a total of 214 subjects, both male and female, studied on 885 subject-nights of sleep. Sleep was interrupted 2,240 times during the REM phase, and these awakenings elicited 1,864 instances of "vivid dream recall," a recall rate of 83.3 percent. When compared to the overall NREM results, the REM period was unquestionably established as the time when the probability of being able to recall a dream is maximal.

My personal conviction was enhanced by one of the earliest studies in which I participated as a subject. I decided to be a subject primarily out of envy; having listened with amazement and awe as many subjects recounted their dreams, I wished to enjoy this experience myself. I learned to attach the electrodes to my own scalp. On the first night I felt like an actor preparing for a performance as I sat in front of the mirror donning my "makeup" of electrodes. I will never forget this "opening night."

After months of arousing others from sleep, I approached the experiment with a definite bias. I knew something of what a dream is, and my own fortuitous morning-after dream-recall experiences had been vivid, long, real, bizarre, and complicated—not just fragmentary images.

A hastily trained medical student, who shall remain nameless, was monitoring the EEG and supervising my arousals. I went to sleep prepared for an exciting night and woke up with a certain urgency and an instantaneous, epic struggle to orient myself. I searched my mind and found nothing but a vague curiosity about what time it was and a feeling that I should recall something. I could remember nothing— but I was not concerned at this point because I knew it is often difficult to remember dreams from the first REM period of the night and that absence of recall occurs, on the average, in one of every five REM awakenings. So I went back to sleep and was suddenly aware of being wrenched from the void once again. This time I could remember nothing except a very, very vague feeling of a name or a person. Disappointed but sleepy, I dozed off again.

The next time I was jolted awake—still unable to recall anything— I began to worry. Why didn't I remember a dream? I had expected to dazzle the medical student with my brilliant recall! After a fourth and a fifth awakening with exactly the same results, I was really upset. What in the world was wrong? I began to doubt the whole REM-dreaming hypothesis. I scoured my memory of past experiments for some flaw, some error by which I might have been biasing the results. Fingers of doubt tickled my consciousness.

I awoke on the sixth arousal with an elusive impression of a man on my mind—and I was in such agony that I actually faked a tiny little tidbit of recall for the medical student. I decided to call it a night. The experience had left me exhausted and extremely puzzled, and I was anxious to look at the polygraphic record of my miserable night. Upon examining the record I discovered, to my utter delight and relief, that the medical student had been mistakenly arousing me in NREM Stage 2—as a result of misinterpreting K complexes for eye movements! Not once had I been awakened during a REM period. The next night, with additional instruction, not to mention a few rather curt reproaches, the medical student hit the REM periods right on the button, and vivid recall flooded my mind with each awakening.

What is a Dream?

Our early conviction was that REM sleep and dreaming were exactly synonymous and that NREM sleep was a mental void—an oblivion. This made it necessary to account for the infrequent, but persistently bothersome dream recall reported from NREM awakenings. Our first interpretation was that the occasional NREM dream report was actually recall of memories persisting from an earlier REM period. This interpretation was swiftly dispatched when investigators demonstrated that occasional dream recall could be elicited from the very first NREM period of the night, before any REM sleep had yet occurred.

In the course of these efforts, we were forced to look much more closely at the reports our subjects were giving us. Many were actually quite ambiguous. It became clear that before we could understand all the sleep-dream relationships, it would be essential to determine exactly what kind of report should be labeled dreaming and what should not. At first, we had assumed that everyone knew what a dream was, so we were a little lax in defining the term precisely. With a little more time and investigation, we came to realize that even if each person's dream experiences were the same, we might not all learn to apply the word "dream" in exactly the same way to exactly the same thing.

Our parents certainly did not tell us what dreams were before the fact. Instead, we produced memories that may or may not have been identified as dreams. Suppose a child says, "Last night I remembered where I lost my water pistol." Although this may have occurred in sleep, it probably will not be recognized as a dream by his parents.

The kinds of experiences we learn to call dreams depend entirely upon the subjective experiences we have had while sleeping and the associations we have made to the experience after awakening. If each person's subjective experience is highly variable, the word "dream" can have very little communicative function. When we asked 500 undergraduate students to define the word "dream," their replies included almost as many differences as similarities. To some the dream action was always a logical progression or sequence; to others there was never a logical occurrence in a dream. Some emphasized the factual, concrete details of their dreams, while others stressed symbolic, abstract imagery. Some students found that dream experience is intensely "real," but others called it strictly "fantasy." To some dreams were natural, to others, supernatural. Some students claimed control over their dreams, while others were merely captives to the dream action. A dream was compared to the television screen or to a vast panorama. Some found dreams to be creative experiences; others found them dull. A dream fulfilled the wishes of some students but frustrated the wishes of others. One defined the dream as "an island of somethingness in a void of nothingness."

As the existence of some NREM dreaming began to be suspected, it became apparent that we could no longer measure dream time by measuring REM time. Researchers became concerned with just how much additional "dreaming" really occurs in NREM sleep and exactly what kind of dreaming this was. We have emphasized the dramatic differences in physiology between REM and NREM sleep, characterizing the brain during REM periods as an "awake" brain. Is it possible that this striking physiological difference does not entail an equally dramatic psychological difference? Such a possibility would require almost wholesale revision of what we assume is a relationship between brain and mind. But to report these REM and NREM recall percentages means very little if we cannot formulate a precise operational definition of the dream.

In the first really important study that closely examined recall from NREM awakenings, the experimenter, David Foulkes, made the need for a precise definition eminently obvious. He counted as dream recall *any* report of mental content, including what might be called "thinking" reports. Subjects, when awakened, were asked, "Was anything going through your mind?" rather than, "Were you dreaming?" Foulkes' approach almost certainly elicited the reporting of additional material that was not specifically labeled as dreaming by the subjects. As a consequence, Foulkes obtained a much higher percentage of "dream recall" from NREM sleep than any previous investigator.

How can we differentiate the "dream" reports from the "thinking" reports? A graduate student of Allan Rechtschaffen, Gene Orlinsky, devised an eight-point scale for judging dream reports:

0. Subject cannot remember dreaming; no dream is reported upon awakening.

1. Subject remembers having dreamed, or thinks he may have dreamed, but cannot remember any specific content.

2. Subject remembers a specific topic, but in isolation; for example, a fragmentary action, scene, object, word, or idea unrelated to anything else.

3. Subject remembers several disconnected thoughts, scenes or actions.

4. Subject remembers a short but coherent dream, the parts of which seem related to each other; for example, a conversation rather than a word, a problem worked through rather than an idea, a purposeful rather than a fragmentary action.

5. Subject remembers a detailed dream sequence in which something happens followed by some consequence, or in which one scene, mood, or main interacting character is replaced by another (different from 3 either in coherence or change in the development of the several parts of the sequence).

6. Subject remembers a long, detailed dream sequence involving three or four discernible stages of development.

7. Subject remembers an extremely long and detailed dream sequence of five or more stages; or more than one dream (at least one of which is rated 5) for a single awakening.

Of 400 NREM recall responses, Orlinsky found that 57 percent fell in the categories 1 through 7. Combining categories 2 through 7, the percent of dreaming was only 46, and percentages declined progressively as fewer categories were included; 6 and 7 together yielded only 7 percent "dream" recall. What emerges very clearly from this study is that the percentage of NREM dreaming is highly sensitive to the criteria used in defining dream recall. This principle helps to explain the differing NREM results among the various studies. The criteria used by Kleitman and myself, although vague, were fairly exclusive. We accepted only "coherent, fairly detailed" descriptions; vague or fragmentary impressions were not recorded as dream recall.

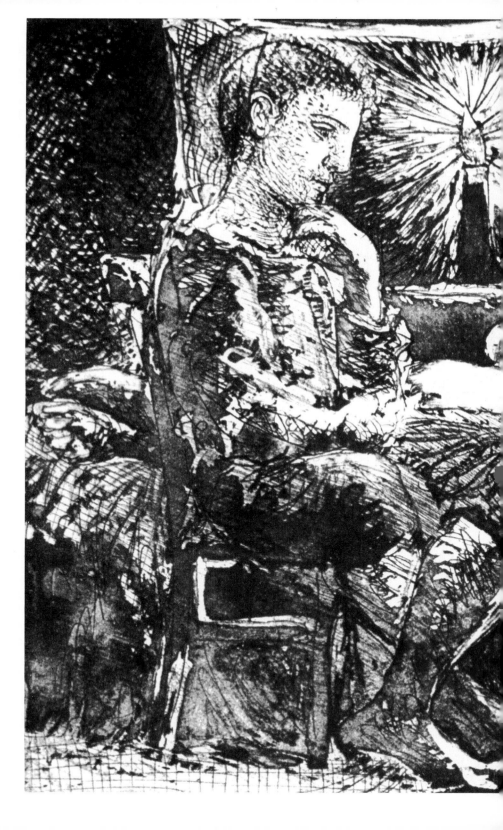

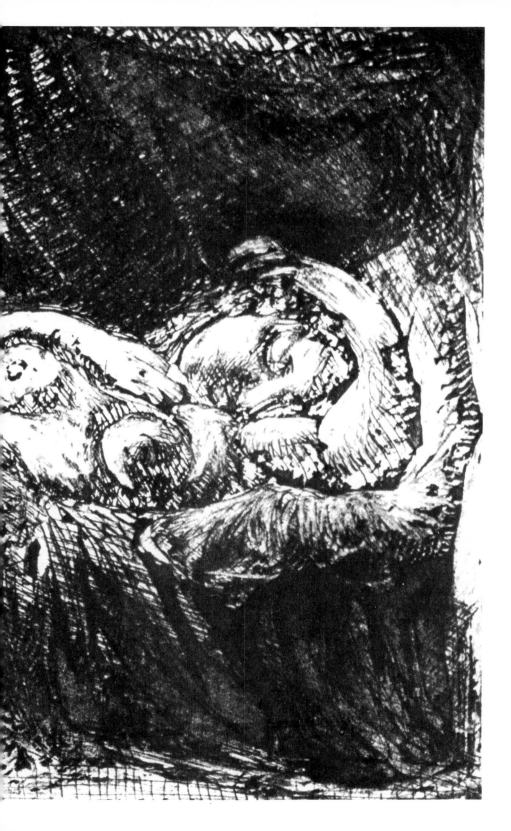

Foulkes, in his 1962 study, defined a dream as "any occurrence with visual, auditory, or kinesthetic imagery" or "any phenomenon lacking such imagery but in which the subject either assumed another identity than his own or felt he was thinking in a physical setting other than that in which he actually was." Not surprisingly, Foulkes obtained a fairly high NREM dream recall rate of 54 percent. Rechtschaffen, in a 1963 study, found that subjects reported some "specific content of mental experience" in 23 percent of NREM awakenings of which he labeled 63 percent as dreaming. Thus only 14.5 percent of his NREM awakenings elicited "dreams."

A number of studies have attempted to compare typical REM and NREM recall. The following examples are from a paper by Rechtschaffen, Vogle, and Shaikun:

> NREM report—"I had been dreaming about getting ready to take some kind of an exam. It had been a very short dream. That's just about all that it contained. I don't think I was worried about it."
>
> REM report (from the same subject awakened later in the night) —"I was dreaming about exams. In the early part of the dream, I was dreaming that I had just finished taking an exam and it was a very sunny day outside. I was walking with a boy who was in some of my classes with me. There was a sort of a . . . a break, and someone mentioned a grade they had gotten in a social science exam, and I asked them if the social science marks had come in. They said yes. I didn't get mine because I had been away for a day." (From "Interrelatedness of Mental Activity During Sleep," in *Archives of General Psychiatry*, 9: 536-37, 1963.)

In spite of the thematic continuity, the second report clearly contains much more of the perceptual vividness and organization that is ordinarily associated with dreaming. Compared with REM recall, NREM mentation is generally more poorly recalled, more like thinking and less like dreaming, less vivid, less visual, more conceptual, under greater volitional control, more plausible, more concerned with contemporary lives, occurring in lighter sleep, less emotional, and more pleasant. The impression is that NREM mentation resembles that large portion of our waking thought that wanders in a seemingly disorganized, drifting, nondirected fashion whenever we are not attending to external stimuli or actively working out a problem or daydream.

Occasionally a NREM awakening will elicit a report that cannot be differentiated from a good REM report; but there is no question that on the average there is a difference between recall from REM and

NREM sleep. In a study by Larry Monroe and his colleagues, two judges were able to state with considerable accuracy whether several hundred reports had been elicited from REM or NREM awakenings.

Two significant facts have emerged from these investigations: REM sleep can no longer be considered exclusively synonymous with dreaming, and NREM sleep is not a mental void.

REM Sleep and Dreaming

In view of our penetrating scrutiny of NREM sleep, perhaps we should take at least one more glance at the REM sleep-dreaming relationship. What does the failure to achieve perfect dream recall from REM period arousals really mean? Does it mean that only four out of five REM periods contain dreams, or does it mean that the subject is dreaming during every REM period but forgets one dream out of five?

Most of us have had the experience of waking from a dream only to have it fade away from our desperately grasping memory. The slightest distraction at this crucial moment—maybe even the sound of the alarm clock—is enough to allow the dream to vanish. Dream recall seems to have an all-or-nothing quality; either we catch the dream and remember most of the story, or we feel it slipping away from us like the fading years of our youth.

On the other hand, the fact that subjects can remember five, ten, sometimes as many as twelve dream episodes from awakenings during a single night is a staggering improvement over the kind of recall that can be elicited by interviewing subjects only in the morning. Our years of experience of having subjects keep dream diaries at home suggest that such recall will always be, except in extremely rare subjects, less than one dream a night. Putting this all together, we feel the most parsimonious conclusion is that dreaming occurs more or less continuously throughout *every* REM period, but in ordinary situations nearly all dreaming is forgotten. In the sleep lab, where the opportunity for remembering dreams is maximized by REM period arousals, the relatively small forgetting rate of about 20 percent seems compatible with the evanescence of dream images. Thus, one of the most solid facts of psycho-physiology is the high probability of dream recall from a REM period arousal.

Time in Dreams

Many people still ask the question, "Are dreams instantaneous?" A dream reported by André Maury in a book called *Sleep and Dreams*, published in 1861, probably played a role in perpetuating this myth. In this dream Maury found himself in Paris during the "reign of terror" following the French Revolution. After witnessing frightful scenes of murder, he was brought before the revolutionary tribunal and confronted by Robespierre, Marat, and other prominent figures of those terrible days. Maury (in his dream) was questioned, condemned, and led to the place of execution surrounded by an immense mob. He climbed onto the scaffold and was bound to the plank by the executioner. The blade of the guillotine fell! Maury felt his head being separated from his body. He then awoke in extreme anxiety and found that the top of his bed had fallen down and had struck his cervical vertebrae in just the way the blade of the guillotine would have struck. Maury reasoned that the awakening stimulus (being struck by the top of the bed) must have initiated the dream, and that all the dream imagery was compressed into the short interval between the initial perception of the stimulus and the awakening.

REM studies have shown, however, that dreams are not instantaneous. Stimuli may modify an ongoing dream but do not initiate it. In our early REM studies we assumed that a dream story unfolds gradually during the REM period. Yet we suspected that awakenings late in a REM period do not elicit total recall; a subject awakened after thirty minutes of REM sleep may remember only the last five minutes with extreme clarity. How could we possibly measure the length of a dream?

One way was simply to count the number of words in the dream report and compare it with the length of the REM period. The eloquence of the dreamer varies according to his mood and memory, the nature of the dream experience, and whether the subject is normally loquacious or taciturn. Nevertheless, we expect that it would take more words to describe a long dream than to describe a short one. In a 1957 study in Kleitman's sleep laboratory we compared the number of words in 126 dream narratives with the objectively measured length of the REM periods from which the subjects had been awakened. Our results showed a positive correlation (for each subject) between the duration of the REM periods and the number of words in the dream narrative. However, when the REM periods were as long as thirty to fifty minutes, the dream narratives were not much longer than those recounted after only fifteen minutes, although the subjects often had the impression they had been dreaming for an unusually long time. This suggests that dream memories may only persist for about fifteen minutes unless they are unusually vivid.

In another series of similar trials, we awakened subjects either five minutes or fifteen minutes after the onset of REM sleep and asked them to designate the correct interval on the basis of the apparent duration of whatever dream material they recalled. A correct choice was made in ninety-two of 111 instances.

Finally, a new technique of inserting external stimuli into the REM period was applied to the problem of the course of time in dreams. Dr. Edward Wolpert and I used a special type of stimulus as a "marker" in the dream. This stimulus was a fine spray of cold water ejected from a hypodermic syringe, and was presented after the subject had been in REM sleep for several minutes. The subject was then allowed to sleep for another few minutes before being awakened and asked to report his dream recall.

We were able to accumulate ten instances in which there was "incorporation" when the stimulus did not awaken the subject, and the interval between the stimulus and the awakening was precisely timed. In these instances, the amount of dream material reported between incorporation and arousal seemed to coincide with the amount of action that could have taken place during an identical length of time in reality.

In most instances, the spray of water was very vividly incorporated into the dream story. A subject who had dreamed he was acting in a play related the following narrative when he was awakened thirty seconds after the old water had been sprayed on his back:

"I was walking behind the leading lady when she suddenly collapsed and water was dripping on her. I ran over to her and water was dripping on my back and head. The roof was leaking. I was very puzzled why she fell down and decided some plaster must have fallen on her. I looked up and there was a hole in the roof. I dragged her over to the side of the stage and began pulling the curtains. Just then I woke up."

The Scanning Hypothesis

Through the years the debate over the so-called scanning hypothesis has become one of the most controversial in which I have ever been involved. Once rapid eye movements had been discovered and related to dreaming, it was very natural to speculate that they had to do with dream imagery—that the sleeping subject's eyes move right or left, up or down, as he "watches" the activity unfolding in his dream.

The first confirmation we gathered was a number of anecdotal instances in which dream recall from awakenings preceded by bursts of exclusively vertical or exclusively horizontal eye movements consisted of dreams that corresponded exactly to the plane of action in the eye movements. In one dream associated with exclusively horizontal eye movements, for example, the subject reported that he was watching a ping pong match.

Our own studies, plus similar studies conducted by Ralph Berger and Ian Oswald in Edinburgh in 1962, showed a high correlation between "active" dreams and active EOGs (i.e. lots of eye movements) and between "inactive" dreams and inactive EOGs. Working with Howard Roffwarg, then of Columbia University, I tested the hypothesis that the oculomotor apparatus in REM sleep behaves as if it were receiving information (sensory input or neuronal barrages) that are, in effect, identical with the sensory input that would elicit the same response in the waking state. (Figure 8)

This series of studies was conducted in a unique sleep laboratory— a rather magnificent apartment overlooking the Hudson River in New York City. A special grant from the National Institute of Mental Health enabled me to defray half the cost of the apartment by converting it into a sleep laboratory with two bedrooms and several work rooms in addition to living quarters for myself and my family. I could work nights without leaving home.

Roffwarg spent the night in a bathroom located between the two bedrooms, while I monitored the emerging EOG patterns on the polygraph. When I detected an eye movement pattern that was distinctive yet fairly simple, I would arouse the subject by means of a buzzer. Then Roffwarg obtained the dream narrative from the subject and attempted to predict the pattern of eye movements on the basis of the dream activity that the subject described. The method can be illustrated by the following dialogue between Roffwarg and a subject describing her dream:

> "Right near the end of the dream I was walking up the back stairs of an old house. I was holding a cat in my arms."
> "Were you looking at the cat?"
> "No. I was being followed up the steps by the Spanish dancer, Escudero. I was annoyed at him and refused to look back at him or talk to him. I walked up as a dancer would, holding my head high, and I glanced up at every step I took."
> "How many steps were there?"
> "Five or six."
> "Then what happened?"
> "I reached the head of the stairs and walked straight over to a group of people about to begin a circle dance."
> "Did you look around at the people?"
> "I don't believe so. I looked straight ahead at the person across from me. Then I woke up."
> "How long was it from the time you reached the top of the stairs to the end of the dream?"
> "Just a few seconds."

On the basis of this interrogation, Roffwarg predicted, "There should be a series of five vertical upward movements as she holds her head

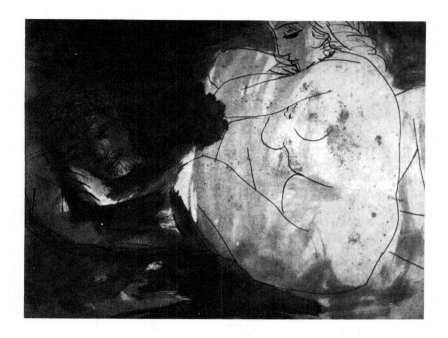

high and walks up the steps. Then there should be a few seconds with only some very small horizontal movement just before the awakening." The associated EOG tracing showed that the temporal sequence and direction of the eye movements were exactly as Roffwarg had predicted they would be.

The difficulty with such studies is that in most instances the eye movements are an incredible mixture not suggesting much of anything. But in a subsequent analysis of the data from this study, we determined that Roffwarg was able to predict quite accurately in a fairly large number of trials. In our minds the matter was settled; we elaborated the "scanning hypothesis"—which has since been referred to somewhat skeptically by Ian Oswald as the "looking-at-pictures hypothesis." Roffwarg and I were convinced that we were able to account for the heightened sense of reality in dreams by hypothesizing that the brain is doing in the REM state essentially the same thing it does in the waking state; a sensory input is being elaborated. In other words, the dream world is "real" precisely because there is no detectable difference in brain activity.

One of the most common objections to the scanning hypothesis was based on the fact that newborn infants show REM periods with lots of eye movements. As far as we can tell, these eye movements are no different from those seen in adult humans. Since it seemed very unlikely that newborn babies were having visual dreams, many people regarded this as evidence that the eye movements were totally unrelated to dreaming. However, the possible lack of a relationship in infants is not crucial proof of a similar lack in adults.

A more critical test of the scanning hypothesis was conducted in persons who were blind from birth. Such persons are known to have dreams which are totally lacking in visual imagery and, hence, no scanning eye movements would be expected to be present in their REM periods. William Offenkranz and Ed Wolpert were the first investigators to study this, and their subject was the blind pianist George Shearing. His sleep was recorded for one night in the same Chicago laboratory where eye movements were originally discovered. He had no eye movements on the EOG and reported only auditory dreams when awakened during REM periods. In this case REM periods were indicated by the typical EEG pattern and by muscle suppression in the EMG.

Oswald and his colleagues studied a group of blind patients and found that in those who were blind from birth no eye movements were detectable. Among those who became blind later in life, Oswald observed eye movements, saw-tooth waves in the EEG, and dreams with visual imagery. Conflicting results reported by subsequent investigators raised some complicated questions, such as whether blind people have a normal corneo-retinal potential (which bears upon the instrumentation used in recording) and whether the eye movements that are detected are really associative eye movements.

Some investigators have attempted to draw conclusions from animal studies. For example, Elliot Weitzman took movies of eye activity during the REM sleep of monkeys (he was fortunate enough to have one monkey that slept with its eyes half open) and thereby documented eye movements very similar if not identical to the scanning movements that occur during wakefulness. Similar results were obtained in the chimpanzee by Jack Rhodes. In addition, there was some evidence that monkeys dream. One group of workers had trained monkeys to press a microswitch with the index finger when they saw a certain visual configuration. They noticed that these monkeys occasionally made the identical finger movements in REM sleep whereas untrained monkeys did not.

But the type of rapid eye movements seen during sleep in the cat tended to undermine the scanning hypothesis. The feline eye movements consist mainly of bursts of small quick jerky movements all in the same plane (quite unlike waking movements). These unique movements, plus the fact that they are related to electrical activity discharged in the brain in bursts of PGO spikes, suggested to some that the eye movements of sleep are programmed according to rules quite different from those in effect during waking visual experience—rules that may not be related to vision at all.

It is interesting that in nearly a decade of argument about the scanning hypothesis, no one attempted to confirm our original findings in human subjects. Finally, just a couple of years ago, two laboratories attempted independent verification of a relationship between dreams and eye movements. They both obtained negative results. However, it was apparent to our group at Stanford that they had not done their dream interrogations in a painstaking manner, and, in addition, they had done relatively few REM period arousals. Because of this, two graduate students, Terry Pivik and Jim Bussel, and I resolved to do a definitive study.

One facet of previous studies that bothered us was the assumption that one ought to be able to predict eye movements with 100 percent accuracy if the scanning hypothesis was valid. The tacit assumption was that 100 percent accuracy would be possible in the waking state when our memories for visual experience would presumably be excellent. We decided to do two studies simultaneously: one in the waking state and one in sleep.

Bussel decorated our laboratory so that it would present a rich visual experience with many objects to look at. Our subjects were asked to sit with their heads in chin rests in order to avoid the complications of head movement. They were told that we were interested in studying recall and instructed to look around the room. The EOG was monitored continuously until a buzzer sounded and the subject was asked to relate what he had been looking at during the last fifteen seconds. Pivik interrogated the subjects and tried to predict the last eye movement. After a series of wakeful studies, the subjects slept in the laboratory, and we repeated the study Roffwarg and I had done in New York.

From this data we made one very startling discovery: There was no significant difference between the results obtained during wakefulness and those obtained during REM sleep periods! Even in the waking state, eye movements could not be predicted with 100 percent accuracy. This demonstrated clearly that one would get negative results even in the waking state if the investigator used only a few trials. For nearly twenty years we, as well as other investigators, had assumed that a high positive correlation would be easy to demonstrate in the waking state—and we were wrong.

Describing Dreams in Process

These and other studies have demonstrated, in our opinion, that dreaming occurs during REM sleep and that the dream is an ongoing experience with a temporal dimension similar to that which occurs in the waking state. Additional evidence to support this contention may be forthcoming as a result of experiments designed to obtain direct verbal descriptions of ongoing REM periods.

Incredible as it may seem, such evidence was recently claimed by a group of Italian investigators. Using a conditioning procedure, these investigators trained ten medical students to free-associate when they heard a white noise during wakefulness. They then attempted to apply the conditioning technique during REM sleep in order to elicit an ongoing report of the dream experience. While monitoring the subjects' sleep via the recording of EEG and EOG, the investigators caused the white noise to occur during REM periods. They reported that verbalization was obtained in all but one instance. But because the investigators failed to record EMG, it is not certain whether their reports arose from REM sleep, NREM Stage 1, or even wakefulness. To my knowledge, this technique has not been replicated successfully.

Louis Aarons has utilized a second technique called evoked sleeptalking. The subjects are trained by means of avoidance-escape conditioning using light and tone stimuli. Vocalization is reinforced by the reduction or removal of stimuli that are unpleasant to the subject. Dr. Aarons has reported responses ranging from snorts and grunts to interjections, phrases, and complete sentences. The technique seems to be lacking in respect to obtaining any ongoing description of dreaming, because the intelligible responses seem to be geared more toward the external stimuli than toward any internal dream experience.

Although neither of these techniques has proved that ongoing verbalization of dream content can be elicited, the possibility that a similar method might prove successful leads to stimulating speculation. How would the dream be described? Would the dreamer narrate the activity? Or would he speak only as one of the characters in the dream fantasy? Is the whole idea as absurd as asking an actor to describe a scene while he is in the midst of acting it out? Would a play-by-play narration of a dream prove that eye movements and the dream are related?

In 1955, Kleitman and I thought that we could tell at what age human beings began to dream by seeing when they began to show rapid eye movements during sleep. Shortly thereafter, we watched newborn babies sleeping in a Chicago nursery and, to our great surprise, saw typical rapid eye movements. A newborn baby cannot tell us whether or not it is dreaming so we will probably never be able to know if dreaming begins this early in life. The existence of REM sleep from birth, plus occasional reports from very young children that seem unquestionably related to dreaming, suggest to us that dreaming may begin long before the child has the verbal ability to describe the dream, or even the intellectual ability to understand the difference between dreaming and waking. A case of dreaming in a very young child was illustrated to me by my own daughter when she was less than two years old. I went into her room one morning before she awoke and saw her eyes moving. Suddenly she said, "Pick me! Pick me!" I woke her and she immediately said, "Oh, Daddy, I was a flower." (Incidentally, such talking does not often occur during REM periods.)

Perhaps it is only in the privacy of our secret thoughts that we can really appreciate the mystery and wonder of the dream world. All-night vigils in the sleep laboratory afford a sleep researcher ample time for private musing about the nightly disembodiment of the self . . . the transformation that allows us to go backward in time to revisit our childhood . . . the transcendent dimension that enables us to visit another planet or another universe . . . the metaphysical element that offers us a glimpse of heaven or hell . . . the wandering of abstract being in the reaches of infinite time. Can it be the same self whose hand reaches out to hush the alarm clock, who yawns and stretches, waking to the cold light of day? Is it possible that we are completely untouched by the vast realm of our dream experiences?

Many of us readily dismiss these nightly excursions into the dream world as second-rate mental activity unworthy of our rational selves. We limit ourselves to the solidity and continuity of the waking world and deny the legitimacy of chance interaction with distant friends, remote places, dead relatives, even gods and demons offered in the dream world. Should we be so anxious to dismiss dreaming—the sole risk-free experience in which we can escape the dreary bondage of time and space?

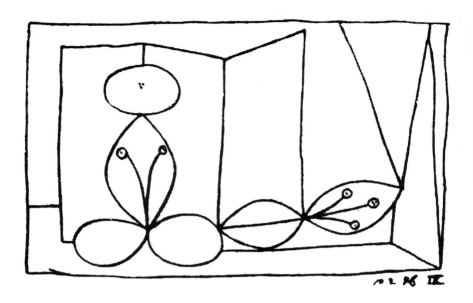

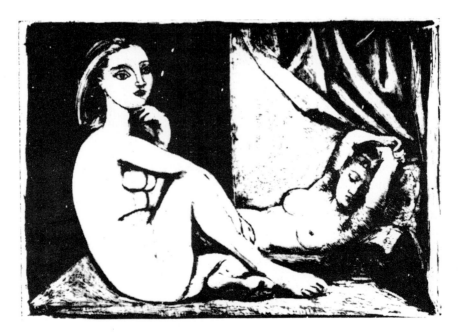

CHAPTER FOUR

THE CONTENT OF DREAMS

"I dreamed I was decapitated. My ribs were picked clean . . . no skin . . . no muscle. My body was cut in half. They didn't know who I was, but I still knew who I was. I wanted to pull myself together, but I couldn't."

THIS DREAM WAS RECOUNTED to Patricia Carrington during a recent study of the dreams of schizophrenics. (From "Dreams and Schizophrenia," in *Archives of General Psychiatry, 26:* 343-50, 1972.) She studied sixty women, thirty schizophrenics and a control group of thirty nonschizophrenics, then compared the dreams of each group on parameters theoretically related to schizophrenia. Dr. Carrington found that in general the schizophrenic dreams gave the impression of an acute state of emergency or stress, while the control dreams depicted everyday, practical concerns. Among the specific themes that she reported as more common to the schizophrenic patient were physical aggression and environmental threats against the dreamer. The patients dreamed of choking, of being impaled, of being closed in by slowly crushing walls.

Although this example gives an indication of the rather horrifying extremes that dreams can achieve and suggests that they might have some diagnostic utility, a consideration of the study as a whole will also bring out some of the difficulties involved in answering the question, "What do people dream about?" For example, "My body was cut in half." How do we know that this is really what the dream depicted, or that it was depicted realistically? Maybe the dream experience was much less traumatic or totally different, but was altered in the process of remembering and reporting. We would not be surprised at such a possibility in a schizophrenic patient, but we must keep in mind that, until we can directly enter the mind of another person, the dream world is entirely private and we cannot be absolutely sure of what transpires there.

Another problem is how to obtain dream samples. REM period awakenings, while they certainly yield greater recall, also alter the dreams by interrupting them before they are completed. Also, the method is too costly in time and energy to be applied readily to large populations. (It might be worth noting that small portable "dream detecting" machines that could be used at home by the subjects are technically feasible.) When spontaneous recall is the only source of dream information, we must assume that most of the dream material is omitted from the sample because it is forgotten. Spontaneous recall was the method used by Dr. Carrington. In addition to the more general problem of forgetting, it is possible that the differences between the schizophrenic and the normal subjects lay not in the dream content *per se*, but in the kind of dream that was spontaneously remembered by each group. Perhaps only the most somber and anxious dreams were recalled by the patients.

Finally, there is the problem of how the tremendous masses of dream data that are often obtained in either kind of study (REM arousals and spontaneous recalls) are summarized and communicated. This task is roughly analogous to summarizing the encyclopedia. What to tabulate, to emphasize? Does one look only at the manifest dream content? Or should interpretive evaluations of the latent content be attempted?

The most objective method for dealing with dream experiences is content analysis. This method is solely concerned with the manifest content of dreams. No interpretations are made and no inferences are drawn about any possible symbolic meaning of the dreams. By far the most extensive attempt to answer the question of what people dream about is the work of Calvin Hall and his associate, Robert Van de Castle. By asking students to write down any dream they remembered, Hall collected thousands of dreams and then applied the method of content analysis in summarizing them. He was eventually able to report that color appeared in 29 percent of the dreams; strangers appeared in

10 percent, somewhat oftener in dreams of women than of men; and so on. Such analysis is affected by the length of the dream, the detail in which it is described, and the idiosyncrasies and personal proclivities of the dreamer.

Several individuals in addition to Hall have used a scientific method for studying dreams. A true pioneer in this area was Mary Whiton Calkins, a psychology instructor at Wellesley College in the 1890s. Introspection was the vogue then, and the papers published by Miss Calkins and her students, Weed and Hallum, are illustrious examples of that method. Miss Calkins said, "It was very simple to record each night immediately after awakening from a dream every remembered feature of it. For this purpose, paper, pencil, candles, and matches were placed close at hand." In spite of the primitive equipment, she and an associate collected 375 dream descriptions, which Miss Calkins proceeded to examine and elucidate in a manner that could still serve as a model of scientific exposition. She found that the majority of the dreams were fairly prosaic; they involved many episodes, people, places, and things that were taken from the current life of the dreamer.

Dr. Fred Snyder, one of the first to do content analysis of REM awakening dreams, arrived at similar conclusions in his paper "The Phenomenology of Dreaming." Snyder found that the most common color in a dream was green, with red fairly close behind. Yellow or blue turned up only half as frequently as green. Snyder concluded, "The broadest generalization I can make about our observations of dreaming consciousness is that it is a remarkably faithful replica of waking life."

Turning to the determinants of dream content, we are confronted by one of the most fascinating questions of all: Is there a supernatural element that determines what we dream about? Before I discuss this topic, I should present my own personal biases; essentially I have none. The existence of extrasensory perception, telepathic communication, or any event that transcends the physical laws of the known universe is certainly not proven; on the other hand, it has not been disproven. Certainly folklore is replete with accounts of prophetic, telepathic, or ESP dreams. Perhaps the efforts to investigate these phenomena are analogous to the task confronting physicists trying to discover whether there are faster-than-light particles.

The most extensive studies of the phenomenon of ESP and its relationship to dreaming are being conducted by Dr. Montague Ullman and his colleagues at the Maimonides Community Mental Health Center in Brooklyn. Results have varied from very poor to fairly good, and it should be noted that until recently studies were not tightly controlled for biasing effects. In a typical study, "The procedures were designed to investigate the hypothesis that telepathic transfer of information from an A (or knowledgeable 'sender') to a sleeping S (subject or 'receiver') could be experimentally demonstrated." The sender was given sealed envelopes containing reproductions of famous paintings and instructed to open one of these during the night after the subject was asleep. The subject was awakened during REM periods, and dream reports were obtained. Several independent judges were later asked to determine whether there was any correlation between the selected painting and the dream report. The design and controls for judging were elaborately prepared to prevent the possibility of bias.

The total number of correlations was not statistically significant, but there were several instances of unique correspondence between the painting and the dream. When the painting was Chagall's "The Drinker" (showing a man drinking from a bottle), the subject reported, "I don't know whether it's related to the dream that I had, but right now there's a commercial song that's going through my mind . . . about Ballantine Beer. The words are, 'Why is Ballantine Beer like an opening night, a race that finishes neck and neck? . . .' "

At a Stanford alumni conference several years ago, an alumnus in the audience asked me if we had conducted experiments in telepathic dreams. We had, but before I recount our experience, just for the record, I should mention that some of my colleagues threatened to drum me out of our professional societies after they heard of the undertaking. They asked me why we were getting mixed up with such nonsense. You just can't win! Anyway, back to our experiment. During the winter term of 1970-71 I had over 600 students enrolled in a course on sleep and dreams and I thought it would be fun and possibly informative if we conducted an experiment whereby the whole class would try to "send a thought" to people who were sleeping in the sleep laboratory. We intended to test the premise that since single individuals might be able to transmit their thoughts into other individuals' dreams once in a while, 600 people all sending the same thought or image at the same time might be able to really blast through.

Six students from the class who felt they might have special "psychic" talents volunteered to be "receivers." These students prepared themselves by going to bed progressively more early so that on the day of the experiment they were able to arrive at the sleep laboratory for the hook-up at about 7 p.m. Meanwhile, the class gathered at 9 p.m. at the Lucille Nixon Elementary School on the campus, one and one-half miles from the sleep lab. Our first problem was what to transmit. We finally selected several commonplace, unambiguous objects—a horseshoe, a banana, a key. We made slides of these objects as well as of the experimental subjects. We communicated by telephone with the sleep lab so we would know when our subjects began REM periods. The scenario went something like this: first, the laboratory technicians would inform us that a subject was having a REM period; then we would flash his picture on the screen to further identify him to those students who did not know him well; the class would decide on an object to concentrate on; and the picture of that object would be projected on the screen. None of the test images that the class "transmitted" were manifested in the dreams of the students sleeping in the laboratory.

In retrospect, there were many things wrong with this cumbersome and difficult experiment. In particular, one difficulty we did not anticipate was that we could not produce absolute synchronicity in 600 minds. It is actually quite hard to concentrate on a horseshoe for an entire minute, and the atmosphere of 600 students at a "happening" created additional handicaps. Finally, showing a slide of the specific student to whom the "message" was being sent was an additional distraction.

As so often happens in this kind of study, we did get one very tantalizing though completely non-statistical result. During the third REM period of one subject, Rod Boone, the class was concentrating on the slide of a horseshoe. After "concentrating" on this image for one minute, we asked the lab technicians to wake Rod and see if he "got the message." There was no mention of shoes or horses, but Rod did give the rather unusual report that he had been dreaming of staring at himself in a mirror! Perhaps our class, or at least its female contingent, had actually concentrated more on the slide of Rod's good-looking face than on the less inspiring horseshoe.

Dream Sequences

Another approach which was made possible by the discovery of REM sleep and the use of laboratory EEG techniques is to examine multiple dreams of a particular subject on a single night. If we arouse a subject in every REM period, we are likely to get four to eight fairly detailed dream reports. Will these dreams be similar or totally different? We might expect the dreams to be similar just because they occur on the same night. However, we occasionally obtain nightly samples where the dreams seem startlingly unrelated and altogether improbable. A sequence from one of my own nights in the sleep lab started out with two hippopotamuses in a millpond, then a taffy pull in the Russian embassy with Premier Khrushchev as one of the pullers;

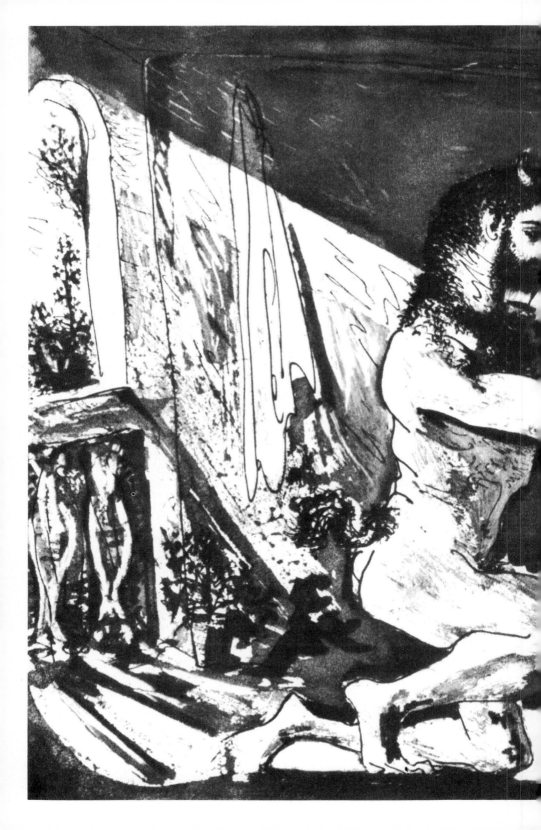

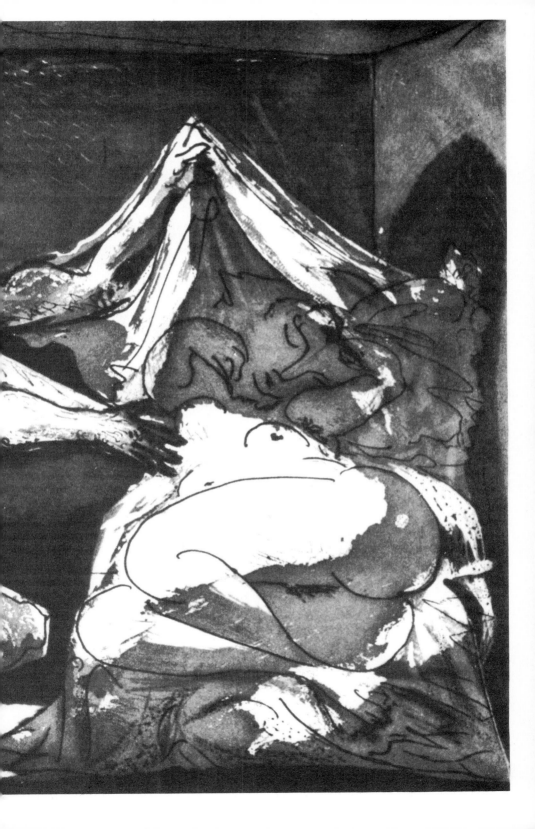

next a motorcycle ride through a wheat field. In the last dream of the night I was at my desk in Riverdale, New York, circa 1959, writing some sort of paper. I have often thought of offering a prize for the most interesting night of dreaming—but such an effort might encourage confabulation.

Is it possible that widely disparate dream episodes are related or linked together by some hidden thought or impulse in the mind of the dreamer? Even on the level of overt dream imagery, the degree and variety of possible relationships are virtually infinite. In the most trivial case, five successive dreams might be said to be related to one another if each one contained the image of a tree or if there were people in each dream. At the other end of the scale, dreams might be related in terms of a complex thematic development or restatement that involves virtually the entire content of each successive dream.

The first study on this topic was done by Dr. Ed Wolpert and me back in 1955-56. By awakening subjects ten to fifteen minutes after the beginning of each successive REM period, we obtained thirty-eight nightly sequences of four to six dreams each distributed among eight adult volunteers. In spite of very careful scrutiny, we did not find the exact duplication of a single dream. Many people say they can wake up from a dream, go back to sleep, and continue the dream. But in our study, no dreams in a sequence were ever perfectly continuous with one taking up just where the preceding one had ended. For the most part, each dream seemed to be a self-contained drama, relatively independent of the preceding or following dreams. Nevertheless, the manifest content of nearly every dream exhibited some obvious relationship to one or more dreams occurring on the same night. In the majority of cases, only contiguous dreams were obviously related.

Some of the relationships seemed quite incidental yet intriguing, as in the following example:

(a) "... I went inside and started going up an escalator. I could see my wife up ahead of me four or five steps. The place was just mobbed. Then we were going down a hallway and I couldn't get to her. There were cakes of ice in the center of the hallway and people just milling in and out, everyone carrying suitcases and things. Then we started up this next escalator, and there was a girl standing beside me. She had a real shabby suitcase. . . ."

(b) "... He was collecting big hunks of watermelon, and I thought I'd get a job helping him, so I started picking them up, and some of them looked more like pieces of ice than they did like watermelon. . . ."

Although the presence of ice illustrates a seemingly trivial relationship between the two dreams, this image, which seems incongruous in both dream narratives, might imply a deeper and more important relationship on the level of the underlying dream thoughts. Thematic correspondence is more extensive in the following narratives elicited from two contiguous REM periods:

(a) "... I went in (a house on a hillside) and I had a feeling that I shouldn't be there or that it was somehow slightly naughty to be in there. Anyway, I was inside and I realized there was a gangster somewhere in the house. There was a third party in the room with us, and we were listening to something going on outside the room. Suddenly we had to escape and we all ... there were three of us, my wife and I and some man, I can't remember who he was but he seemed to belong ... and we had to get away, so we jumped out the window. Then we got into the car and I yelled to this guy, for some reason, that I ought to drive. He didn't know how to drive our car, but there was something about him—like he was a movie hero or something—and he was taking over. He jumped behind the wheel, and he went roaring up the hill. Someone shot at us out the window as we ran off. ..."

(b) "It started out with me telling somebody about a murderer. The murderer was supposed to be in this house. I was telling two detectives a rather lengthy story about this gruesome murder. The idea was to lock them in this house with the murderer so they'd catch him. And my wife, or some woman who was somehow related to me, was supposed to leave. So she went outside and I locked them in. Just as I finished locking them in the house it occurred to me that this was a trick, and the murderer was this woman, and she was having me lock the detectives in the house so she could get me. Just as I went running down the porch stairs this horrible knowledge dawned on me. I ran out into the yard and was kind of looking at the house. It was an old house on a hill. The yard was kind of roundish. Suddenly she jumped out of the bushes and began running at me. She looked horrible. She was going to push me off the cliff—part of the hill was a cliff—or kill me somehow. Just before she got to me she changed into a tiger— a tigress. At that moment I woke up crying out."

In each of these dream narratives, a house on a hill is the locale, and the dreamer leaves the house because of some danger. A gangster appears in the first dream and a murderer in the second. However, there seems to be a reversal of circumstances between the two dreams. In the first the danger is within the house, and a safe exit is made by the dreamer and his companions. But in the second the danger is on the outside, and the dreamer is unable to escape but must awaken in terror.

Another longer sequence revealed a very complicated scheme of relationships through four contiguous dreams. The dreamer seemed to be at the center of a kind of classical tragedy, in which those elements of strength which appear in the first dream are the very forces that vanquish him in the fourth. Although the dreams themselves are too long and detailed to be useful here, a summary of the elements will show the skein of interrelationships.

(a) He dreams about a woman whom he has successfully thwarted, and to whom he says: "Let me see your trump card. Let me just look at you." He looks her in the face.

(b) Another man shoots a woman in the back and the dreamer becomes afraid and runs.

(c) The dreamer is seduced by a woman and made to behave passively. A third woman helps to "instruct" him how to make love. Later, he cuts himself on a razor which he has left on a chair and forgotten. The dream ends in a sequence where he is instructing a young boy about the traditionally masculine activity of hunting.

(d) He is playing cards, seated with two women at a bridge table. When he senses something puzzling, he looks at his cards. His are the wrong kind of cards.

As far as we know, the only available method of gathering this type of dream sequence material is the practice of awakening subjects during the REM period. However, this method has at least two important limitations. First, since one can never be certain in advance exactly how long an individual REM period will last, the awakening must occur fairly shortly after the REM period onset. An unknown amount of material is lost because the dream is prevented from reaching its natural termination. Secondly, the procedure of the awakening undoubtedly disturbs the dream pattern. Not only is the dream abruptly and unnaturally terminated, but a series of events, namely the awakening, the description of the dream, and the handling of the recording apparatus, might induce a spurious relationship of one dream to another. An example of this was vividly demonstrated in a dream sequence that occurred when Charles Fisher and I were studying the effects of REM sleep deprivation.

In this study, we hoped to learn whether dreaming represents an oral drive experience. If so, we could possibly substitute eating for dreaming by waking the subject as soon as a REM period started and by feeding him during each of these awakenings. This theory was not substantiated by our experiment—but one of the dream sequences illustrated how the arousal and the interaction between the subject and the investigator can become incorporated into subsequent dreams.

The first subject we tested told us his favorite food was banana cream pie. Mrs. Fisher baked a delicious, creamy confection and we took it to the lab to begin the experiment. Following the usual procedure in REM deprivation studies, we waited until there were several eye movements, then awakened the subject, who reported a short fragment of a dream about walking down a street in Greenwich Village. He ate his first piece of banana cream pie with great gusto and commented, "What a way to do research!" He went back to sleep, began another REM period about an hour later, recalled another dream fragment when we awoke him, and again ate his pie with relish. After three awakenings, three minute dreams, and three pieces of pie, the fourth arousal elicited the following dream: "I was having a cup of coffee and a cigarette." He ate his fourth piece of banana cream pie with a little less enthusiasm and commented, "I always have coffee and a cigarette at the *end* of meals." Describing the fifth dream fragment, he said, "I was given some spaghetti, but I was scraping it off the plate into a garbage can." He ate his fifth piece of pie with obvious reluctance and left the crust. In the sixth dream fragment he reported, "Dr. Dement, I dreamed I was feeding *you* banana cream pie!"

When Rechtschaffen included NREM awakenings in a study of dream sequences, he discovered a thematic continuity in which the vivid perceptual activity of the REM period appeared as a kind of reflection in the NREM awakening and was then transformed into a dream theme in the next REM period. In other words, the NREM dreaming may have some significance in determining the relationship of successive REM dreams. In Rechtschaffen's study some continuity continued throughout the night in both REM and NREM sleep.

We cannot account for what determines thought processes. In wakefulness it is often nothing more than attending to the environment. We know what we would be thinking about during a football game, for example, but with less stimulation our minds can wander in the most improbable directions following random thoughts. Sometimes we have an experience that persists in our consciousness; we have just heard news of the death of a good friend or close relative. The sadness, the upset, the loss stays with us all day and determines our thoughts. Perhaps a similar process takes place in dreaming and other mental activity during sleep; if some significant event has occurred, we will think about it and dream about it one way or another all night long.

This kind of process is found in the dreams of a subject spending his first night in the sleep laboratory. A naïve subject, seeing the rather impressive equipment and having wires attached to his head, will feel extremely anxious; something is going on that has to do with electricity. In a study I did with Ed Kahn and Howard Roffwarg, we looked at first-night dreams and found that about one-third of them clearly depicted the laboratory situation and the feelings of the subject. This figure dropped to about 10 percent on later nights when the subject was confident that the equipment was not dangerous.

Here is an excerpt from a first-night dream: "I dreamed I was lying here and something went wrong so that any second I was going to be electrocuted. I wanted to tear the wires off, but suddenly realized that my hands were tied. I was very relieved when you woke me up."

If dreams occurring on later nights reflect the laboratory situation, they are usually much less fearful: "[I dreamed] you came in and told me there was a big party going on next door. We decided to call it a night and go to the party. After the electrodes were off, I put on a tuxedo and went over. A whole bunch of people were dancing and I saw this girl standing in the corner...."

Herman Witkin and Helen Lewis studied the effects of presleep stimuli on dreaming by showing movies to their subjects before they went to sleep in the laboratory. One of the movies was a color film depicting childbirth; another showed the circumcision rite of a primitive tribe; and the third was a pleasant travelogue. The experimenters found only veiled references to the first two movies in the dreams. In some instances, they reported that the dreams appeared to be influenced by insignificant details that the subjects did not even remember having seen in the movies. From these results, Witkin and Lewis proposed the tentative conclusion that insignificant events may be more influential in determining dream content than significant events. Of course, it is always difficult to assess the "significance" of certain experiences, particularly across the generation gap. In other words, the childbirth and circumcision movies may have seemed more traumatic to the experimenters than they really were for their younger subjects.

Stimuli: External and Internal

We have shown that, in general, stimuli do not instigate dreams. But if a stimulus happens to coincide with a REM period, can it influence the dream content? Anecdotal literature is replete with examples: someone who dreamed of thunder awakened to hear the clatter of

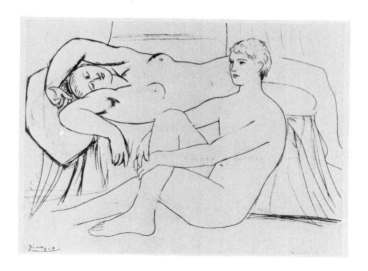

horses hooves on the pavement; someone who dreamed of a roaring conflagration awakened to find a candle flickering by his bed.

One of the first studies of the relationship between stimuli and dream content which utilized the new technique of REM period awakenings was conducted by Dr. Ed Wolpert and myself in 1958. In this study we inserted three different, relatively non-specfic stimuli into REM periods. The first stimulus was a 1,000 cps pure tone sounded for five seconds at a level slightly below the awakening threshold of REM sleep. The second was a flashing 100-watt lamp placed where it would shine directly into the sleeper's face. The final stimulus was a fine spray of cold water ejected from a hypodermic syringe. From our discussion of time in dreams in Chapter Three, you will remember that this was especially effective. The stimulus was presented after the characteristic change in the EEG and rapid eye movements had signaled the start of a REM period. If the stimulus did not awaken the subject, he was allowed to sleep for another few minutes before being awakened and asked to report his dream recall.

The dream reports were subsequently examined to determine whether the stimulus had been incorporated into the dream. Incidence of stimulus incorporation varied from 42 percent for the spray of water to 23 percent for the light flashes and 9 percent for the pure tone. It should be noted that the water spray, as common sense would tell us, was most easily recognized in the dream reports. Nonetheless, there appeared to be a kind of hierarchy of incorporation. In addition, although a stimulus was presented fifteen times during periods of

NREM sleep, no REM periods were initiated and no dreams were recalled on these occasions.

Since the time of this early study, several investigators, with various objectives in mind, have conducted studies using external stimulation. Ralph Berger used spoken names that were either emotionally significant or neutral to the subjects. The names were presented below the threshold of arousal during REM sleep. Berger reported an incorporation rate of about 54 percent but no differences in incorporation between emotional and neutral stimuli. Furthermore, he concluded that perception of external stimuli occurs during REM sleep but that the origin of the stimuli is perceived as a part of the dream.

Vincenzo Castaldo and Philip Holzman used recordings of the subject's own voice and of other voices as their stimuli. When the subject's own voice was played, the principal figure of the dream was more active, assertive, independent, and helpful. When another's voice was played, the main figure was unequivocally passive.

Hoping to provide a conclusive demonstration of the effects of particular stimuli on dream content, several freshmen in my Sleep and Dreams class of 1970-71 conducted an exhaustive study. (The results of this study were recently published in the *Stanford Quarterly Review*, Winter 1972. Other studies done by this class will appear in this undergraduate publication, and I highly recommend it for further reading.) This study involved elaborate procedures and statistical analysis and independent judges were used to rate the amount of incorporation of each stimulus.

The students chose as their stimuli taped recordings of twelve very familiar and evocative sounds such as a rooster crowing, a steam locomotive, a bugle playing reveille, a dog barking, traffic noise, and a speech by Martin Luther King Jr. The subjects were monitored according to the usual procedures, and the sound tape was played starting at approximately ten seconds after the onset of a REM period.

The students found that the sound influenced dream content in 56 percent of the recorded dreams; the locomotive sound was the most effective and traffic noise the least. A strong incorporation of the steam locomotive is illustrated by the following report:

"I dreamed I was riding in a train. I was driving the engine, and the train was in Branner, and right close to the engine there was this pit. It was about two or three stories long, and it was still open, and the train kind of chugged down into it, and it was real scary. I was dreaming the whole time. When I was going into the pit . . . it was amazing because there were some people at the top of the pit watching me go down."

Another area of interest is the effect of internal stimuli on dreams. There are many anecdotal accounts of explorers who were lost and starving and dreamed of sumptuous meals. But Ansel Keys, in his detailed study of the effects of prolonged starvaton during World War II, kept track of the dreams of his starving volunteers and found no particular increase in dreams about food and eating. Ed Wolpert and I attempted to determine the effect of thirst on dreams. Three subjects on five occasions completely restricted their intake of fluids for twenty-four hours or longer before sleeping in the laboratory. On each occasion the subjects reported that they were extremely thirsty when they went to bed, and twice the thirst had reached the point at which the subject had dry lips and was unable to salivate. Fifteen dream narratives were obtained under these conditions, and in no case did the dream content involve an awareness of thirst or descriptions of actual drinking. Five of the dreams, however, contained elements that seemed clearly related to the theme of thirst and drinking:

(a) "I was in bed and was being experimented on. I was supposed to have a malabsorption syndrome."

(b) "I started to heat a great big skillet of milk. I put almost a quart of milk in."

(c) "Just as the bell went off, somebody raised a glass and said something about a toast. I don't think I had a glass."

(d) "While watching TV I saw a commercial. Two kids were asked what they wanted to drink and one kid started yelling, 'Coca-Cola, Orange, Pepsi,' and everything."

(e) "I was watching a TV program, and there was a cartoon on with animals like those in the Hamm's beer advertisement."

I was a subject for this thirst study and recall waking up feeling immediately and painfully thirsty. On one occasion I thought I heard raindrops falling on the window. When I looked outside, I saw the full moon and the stars. I think my desire for water was so great that I momentarily hallucinated the raindrops.

Studies of thirst and hunger seem to answer, at least as a first approximation, the question raised by Freud's wish-fulfillment hypothesis, that the dream represents an attempt to fulfill a wish. In Freud's theoretical framework, the wish was not evident in the manifest content, but was in some way disguised. We can see no reason for disguising the wish in the case of thirst. The psychoanalyst would postulate that this wish is fulfilled in a disguised manner when some seemingly unrelated dream event is in fact a symbolic representation of drinking water. This is very difficult to prove or disprove, because even the analysis of the dream by the method of free association would not provide crucial evidence. If the subject were thirsty, very likely his associations to the dream (or to virtually anything for that matter) would eventually drift toward the subject of water and drinking. The fact that dreams may be interpreted or understood in terms of wish-fulfillment simply is not direct proof that the content occurred for the express purpose of fulfilling the wish.

A salient feature of dreaming is often our total inability to exercise control over the events of the dream. Nonetheless, I have found that many of the students and alumni we have questioned report they are able to control dream content on occasion. The fact that nearly every dream takes unexpected and seemingly random jumps and sudden departures makes these occasional episodes of control all the more interesting.

Drugs can exert an influence on the content of dreams, but this effect seems to be somewhat indirect. We know that the chronic use of barbiturates, monoamine oxidase inhibitors, alcohol, or reserpine (rawoulfia serpentina) can lead to nightmares; but in every case the really frightening nightmares occur following withdrawal of the drug when REM sleep is tremendously intensified.

The intensity of brain stem activity and activation of primitive emotional circuits may be what really determine the sense of dread in dreams. It should be noted that an affective response is no always related to the content of the dream. For example, when approaching a door in a dream one may suddenly experience an incredible dread of opening the door and seeing whatever is on the other side, although the response has nothing to do with the specific visual content. Once the dread is present, it may influence what subsequently appears in the dream. In other words, emotion may sometimes determine what we see, rather than always the other way around.

Many people feel that the tapestry of the dream is woven exclusively from the virtually infinite number of sensory images experienced on the preceding day. However, a study by Roffwarg and his colleagues suggests that elements of the dream are derived from sources other than the previous day's experience. These investigators permitted subjects to experience only the color red while awake. They wore red goggles that filtered all light except a narrow range of frequencies in the red band of the visible spectrum. When subjects saw only red in the day, the red in their dreams increased; but blue, green, and other colors continued to appear in dreams after a week of experiencing only red during the day. Additional evidence is provided by the dream diary of a young man who was paralyzed in a college football game several years ago. Although some of his dreams include experiences in which he is paralyzed and in his wheelchair, others include experiences in which he is able to walk and play football again, and still others include both physical conditions.

Mental activity at the onset of sleep provides another key to determinations of dream content. H. Silberer described a phenomenon in which at the onset of sleep there seems to be a transformation from conceptual and abstract thinking to a kind of perceptual thinking. One can often observe this by waking a subject immediately after he goes to sleep. One subject said, "I was thinking of my mother-in-law's visit, and all of a sudden I saw a big stack of books starting to fall over." Such images appear to be a symbolic representation of a preceding (presumably wakeful) thought, and this is one of the few instances in which transformations are readily observable.

The onset of sleep appears to be related to REM sleep, particularly in regard to the visual imagery and myoclonic jerks. In newborn infants the onset of sleep is REM sleep, and some vestige of this may stay with us throughout life. In normal adults the first REM period is usually removed from the waking world by sixty minutes or more of NREM sleep, allowing ample time for the random thought process to depart from the wakeful setting and mental content. Rechtschaffen's evidence shows that the later in the night the dream is elicited, the less relationship it bears to the events of the previous day and the contemporary world, and the more relationship it bears to the events of childhood. Later dreams seem to draw more and more upon stored images.

Associations that occur as time passes in sleep may be similar to this intrusion of visual images at the onset of sleep. They are not real perceptions, but visual thoughts or brief fragmentary images raised to a more intense level. Even if these associations were to progress as they do in the waking state, by the time the first REM period arrived they would be so far removed from the thought at the onset of sleep that there would be no way of recognizing the connection unless we could trace every step of the circuitous route of the thought process. Even so, it is unlikely that such a connection could be made in the absence of an intense preoccupation acting as a link.

Can we dream of things we have never seen? I would say yes—if they are recombinations, inversions, or resemblances of things we have seen, or if they are things we could draw or conceive of while awake. It is hard to say whether we could dream of something that we could not even conceive of in the waking state.

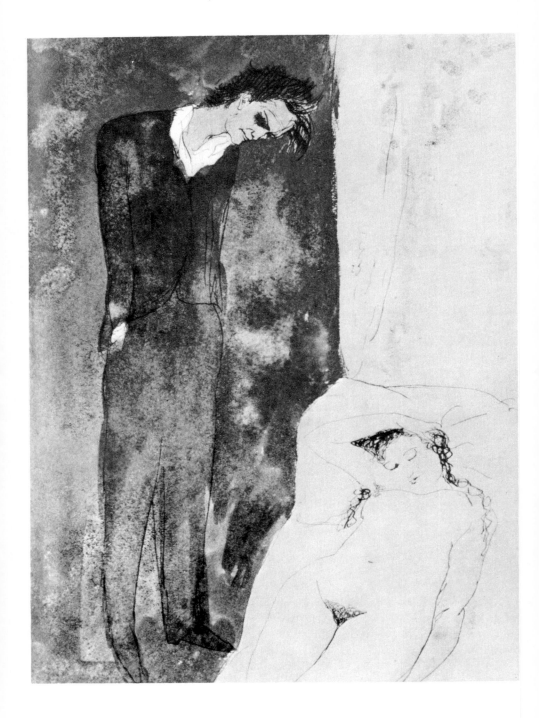

CHAPTER FIVE

SLEEP DISORDERS AND TREATMENT

The first time I went to a doctor for my insomnia, I was twenty-five—that was about thirty years ago. I explained to the doctor that I couldn't sleep; I had trouble falling asleep, I woke up many, many times during the night, and I was tired and sleepy all day long. As I explained my problem to him, he smiled and nodded. Inwardly, this attitude infuriated me—he couldn't possibly understand what I was going through. He asked me one or two questions: Had any close friend or relative died recently? Was I having any trouble in my job or at home? When I answered no, he shrugged his shoulders and reached for his prescription pad. Since that first occasion I have seen I don't know how many doctors, but none could help me. I've been given hundreds of different pills—to put me to sleep at night, to keep me awake in the daytime, to calm me down, to pep me up— have even been psychoanalyzed. But still I cannot sleep at night.

Sleep Apnea

FOR NEARLY THIRTY YEARS this man had lived in the tortured existence of the insomniac. This insidious problem creeps into every aspect of the sufferer's life. Every waking moment becomes filled with anxiety. "Will I be able to sleep tonight?" Every sleepless night he wonders: "How can I make it through another day?" Sleepiness and fatigue make even the simplest task an overwhelming effort.

Imagine living this nightmarish existence for nearly thirty years. Is it conceivable that modern medicine offers no relief to this man? He had tried all the time-honored remedies, from barbiturates to warm milk, yet his sleeplessness continued unabated. Finally, this patient heard about the Stanford University Sleep Disorders Clinic and came to us in the spring of 1972 as his last resort.

At that time, we thought we had an understanding of insomnia pretty well in hand, but our confidence proved premature. The man's medical records ruled out any secondary causes of the insomnia, and for a time we were at a complete loss. Fortunately, my colleague, Dr. Christian Guilleminault, latched onto a critical factor in the patient's history, one that gave us the clue to the cause of his insomnia. Interestingly enough, this crucial point was nothing more than the patient's report that he snored at night, and quite loudly, according to his wife. Due to Guilleminault's fortuitous insight, we added the measurement of respiration to our routine all-night sleep recordings.

We could not contain our astonishment when we found that the patient breathed *only when he was awake*. Watching the chart, paper unfold, we stared open-mouthed as the patient fell asleep and stopped breathing for nearly one hundred seconds. Then, huge scribbles were inked on the respiration chart as he awoke to take gasping breaths into his air-starved lungs. This patient was unable to breathe and sleep at the same time. He had to wake up hundreds of times in order to get enough oxygen to survive the night.

Although we were the first to describe this illness in insomnia, it had been noted in 1965 in patients complaining of *too much* sleep, by Henri Gastaut of Marseilles. This condition is called *sleep apnea* (apnea means cessation of respiration) and because it has been known, in one form at least, since 1965, we are familiar with the associated physiological changes. (Figure 9) The change from wakefulness to sleep affects the central nervous control of breathing (respiratory center) so that it abruptly ceases to function. This causes the diaphragm and the intercostal muscles, muscles essential for breathing, to become immobile. In this phase of the apnea, which lasts for fifteen to thirty seconds, the amount of oxygen in the red blood cells falls to an extremely low level and the carbon dioxide in the blood rises, signaling that air is needed by the body. Eventually the change in these blood gas levels stimulates the respiratory center and the respiratory muscles begin to function again. However, the lungs do not fill because the throat has collapsed, choking off the flow of air. In other words, although respiratory effort is initiated by the diaphragm and intercostal muscles, the sleeping patient still cannot move air through his airway. The collapse of the throat is apparently due to an exaggeration of the muscular relaxation that normally accompanies sleep. After about sixty to one hundred airless seconds, the extreme blood gas changes have an arousing effect, the patient wakes up, tone returns to the throat muscles, and the patient takes a series of cacophonous choking respirations. As a rule, the arousal lasts only a few seconds as the blood gases normalize, the patient immediately returns to sleep, and the cycle is repeated.

Most people with sleep apnea complain of hypersomnia—sleeping too much at night, falling asleep and being very sleepy during the day. In view of the hundreds of arousals that occur each night, it is little wonder that these patients are sleepy in the daytime. Apparently these patients are so habituated to their illness that they are completely unaware of the fact that they may awaken as many as 500 times during the night; they are also oblivious of the fact that they cannot breathe and sleep at the same time. The patients with sleep apnea who complain of insomnia, on the other hand, appear not to habituate to the arousals and do not return to sleep immediately after the apnea. It is possible that individuals who think their sleep is entirely normal may also have sleep apnea. They may be somewhere in between the insomniac and the hypersomniac and be completely insensitive to their problem. About one-third of the sleep apnea patients who have come to our clinic complain of insomnia and the rest of hypersomnia.

At present we do not know how or when this illness begins. Some people think that it may be present at birth and may even account for the sudden infant death (crib death) syndrome. However, the mean age of the patients is fifty-two years; the youngest was thirty-eight.

Treatment of sleep apnea is still in the experimental stage. In addition to various drugs that are being studied, perhaps the most promising treatment for many cases is a surgical procedure that allows the patient to breathe through a tube inserted into his air-way through a hole in his throat.

Unfortunately, only a handful of American physicians are aware of the existence and ramifications of sleep apnea. In fact, the whole area of disordered sleep, while it includes the most prevalent of all illnesses, is still the most obscure. Millions of people say they cannot sleep, and how many know the real reason for their sleeplessness? Recent discoveries in clinical sleep research have shown that conventional treatments for these complaints may actually be harmful to the patients. By highlighting a few more primary sleep disorders, as I have done with sleep apnea, I hope to convey some understanding of the complex and serious nature of these problems.

Narcolepsy

A woman starts to laugh. She topples as if clubbed and her flaccid body seems almost to bounce as it smashes to the ground. A man is playing softball. He is at bat. He takes a terrific cut at the ball and goes suddenly limp; the bat drops from his hands. His body slumps and falls. Still other people report that they cannot hunt because the surprise of seeing birds flush causes them to drop the gun and fall to their knees. It is almost impossible for many people to spank their children, especially if they are angry.

These sudden attacks of complete or partial muscular paralysis precipitated by strong emotion are known collectively as *cataplexy*. They are part of a syndrome of disordered sleep called *narcolepsy*. Although the major symptom of narcolepsy is the periodic occurrence of overwhelming sleepiness during the day, it is cataplexy that is crucial to making the diagnosis since daytime sleep attacks by themselves could also suggest several other illnesses.

During cataplectic seizures, the patient remains fully awake and aware of what is going on around him. Some patients may have hundreds of these attacks in a single day, while others may have only one or two a month. Since the attacks are characteristically triggered by strong emotion, the number of cataplectic seizures is, to some extent, a function of the patient's ability to control his emotions—to become a robot. The narcoleptic patient sails between Scylla and Charybdis. If he allows himself unbridled, spontaneous emotional expression, he will be battered by repeated falls; if he rigidly controls himself, he will cease to be fully alive.

Most of the day the narcoleptic is normally alert. Sleepiness comes in sudden waves and often claims its victim no matter how hard he fights. Sometimes the drowsiness catches him unaware and he falls asleep without realizing. If this happens in a speeding automobile . . .

The things that usually make us all a little drowsy—lying in the sun, a heavy meal, boring lectures—will bring on sleep attacks in narcoleptics. However, they may also fall asleep in very unlikely situations. I believe the most unusual account in my experience was a narcoleptic lady who told me she once fell asleep twenty feet under water—while scuba diving. Falling asleep in the middle of lovemaking is not terribly unusual for narcoleptics.

In addition to cataplexy and sleep attacks, narcoleptic patients often have two other symptoms—sleep paralysis and hypnagogic hallucinations. Sleep paralysis is when the patient suddenly realizes he cannot move just as he is about to fall asleep. This symptom also appears in otherwise normal individuals. For example, in a casual survey of 1,200 Stanford students in our Sleep and Dream courses, we found that approximately 50 percent reported having had at least one episode of sleep paralysis, although only a very small number complained of "abnormal" sleep.

Hypnagogic hallucinations are vivid, often frightening dreams that occur at the onset of sleep. The dream events are often smoothly continuous with the immediately prior waking events. An example of this type of dream occurred recently in the Sleep Disorders Clinic. We were about to begin a clinical recording on a presumptive narcoleptic. I made a final check of the electrode lead wires in the jack-box and left the bedroom. The patient immediately fell asleep and dreamed that I had come back into the room with a scalpel to cut off his ear—my new treatment for sleepiness!

The syndrome of narcolepsy, particularly the symptom of cataplexy, was very puzzling to physicians for many years. Some doctors tried to treat the illness by psychotherapy, thinking the symptoms were neurotic. Understanding came suddenly in 1962, thanks to modern sleep research. Out of sheer curiosity, Allan Rechtschaffen, Charles Fisher, and I did some all-night sleep recording in a few narcoleptic patients. To our great surprise, these patients began a night of sleep, not with the NREM phase in the conventional manner, but with the REM phase. They went immediately from wakefulness into REM sleep. This finding stimulated Rechtschaffen, George Gulevich, and me to study daytime narcoleptic sleep. We confirmed what we had suspected from our previous nighttime study. The narcoleptic sleep was an attack of REM sleep!

This knowledge also helped to explain the symptom of hypnagogic hallucinations. We could understand these hallucinations as the vivid dreams associated with attacks of REM sleep. In addition, our findings offered an explanation of the mysterious attacks of cataplexy.

A powerful inhibitory influence paralyzes the arms, legs, and trunk of the normal sleeper in each and every REM period. It is this paralysis that enables us to have vivid dreams and yet remain asleep. If the intense activity of the dreaming brain were not blocked at the spinal cord level by a strong inhibitory influence, the sleeper would quite literally leap out of his bed. The inhibition must be very strong because it is part of an absolutely essential balance of power in the mechanics of REM sleep—the frenzied turbulence of the brain perfectly balanced against the smothering inhibition of the spinal cord. All that gets out is an occasional twitch. Obviously, this inhibiting paralysis must never erupt during wakefulness. Imagine primitive man trying to escape a saber-toothed tiger and having an attack of cataplexy. There must be some other regulatory mechanism which holds the inhibitory force completely in check during wakefulness, except in the patient with narcolepsy. In such patients, the inhibitory process does break out, often felling its victims in mid-stride like a scythe going through a wheat field.

If the cataplectic attack is unusually long, it may develop into a full-blown REM period with dreaming and rapid eye movements. Every night when the narcoleptic goes to sleep, the first thing that occurs is paralysis (cataplexy). The other REM processes soon follow, but if the narcoleptic patient should try to move before he is actually asleep, he will realize that he cannot. This is sleep paralysis.

Although a great deal of progress has been made in terms of charac-terizing and interpreting the symptoms of narcolepsy, little is known about the precise pathological mechanism. Evidence for a genetic basis comes from the concentration of the disorder in certain families. Nar-colepsy has a characteristic age of onset, usually the decade between ten and twenty years. Although the illness may begin after thirty, it rarely begins after the age of forty. No one has as yet had the opportu-nity to study narcoleptic patients objectively at the immediate onset of the symptoms. At Stanford we are following the children of our narco-leptic patients very closely in an attempt to provide answers to the de-velopmental mysteries.

Contrary to popular belief, narcolepsy is *not* rare. In a special preva-lence study conducted by our clinic, we found that approximately 2,000 persons in the San Francisco Bay area have narcolepsy. We estimate that the illness may affect as many as 100,000 people in the United States. In a modern industrialized and urbanized country, the hazards to persons suffering from narcolepsy are often life-threatening. In our own clinical material, 40 percent of the narcoleptic patients reported one or more serious accidents resulting from sleepiness while driving. One patient, a fireman, reported a cataplectic attack that occurred while he was climbing a ladder to a burning building.

At present there is no cure for narcolepsy, and no complete remis-sion of symptoms has ever been reported. A group of drugs called tri-cyclic antidepressants are usually effective in controlling cataplexy. Methylphenidate (Ritalin), a non-amphetamine stimulant, may be pre-scribed to diminish the sleep attacks. However, the only hope for a really effective treatment in narcoleptics (and patients with other sleep disorders as well) is the research now going on in basic sleep laborato-ries around the world. We must unravel this inhibitory process, find out exactly where it comes from, what controls it, what sets it off. A major share of the resources of the Stanford Sleep Laboratories is devoted to this problem.

Sleepwalking and Related Disorders

Curiously enough, there are sleep disorders where the most severe effects are not seen in the patients. Somnambulism (sleepwalking), enuresis (bed-wetting), and *pavor nocturnus* (night terrors) occur almost exclusively in young children, but it is their parents who suffer, worrying about the "psychological" significance of the episodes. Yet, on the morning after, the children are blissfully ignorant of the fact that anything unusual has happened.

Laboratory studies have shown that these episodes arise in the oblivion of the first deep Stage 4 sleep of the night and are generally associated with body movements and intense autonomic activation. No one really knows the cause of these disturbances, but two hypotheses have been offered by Dr. Roger Broughton. First, he suggests that the episodes may represent the expression of emotional conflicts that are repressed during wakefulness, but are allowed to occur because some psychic barrier is lowered in sleep. On the other hand, he suggests that the attacks may be caused by some purely physiological abnormality that arises in a "psychological void."

The most dramatic and disturbing of the disorders is the night terror: a blood-curdling screech breaks the stillness of the night, bringing distraught parents sprinting to their child's bedside. The dazed and groggy child, his heart racing in response to the unseen night terror, cannot tell his parents what is wrong—he has completely forgotten whatever caused this banshee wail to interrupt his sleep. In no time at all, however, the little child is sound asleep again. In spite of the nocturnal terrors, the youngster is totally normal during the day.

These NREM sleep disturbances tend to run in families. In fact, one of our patients claimed that his entire family—aunts, uncles, parents, siblings—are sleepwalkers. He recounted this amusing story of a family reunion at Christmas time: he awoke one night to find himself surrounded by all his sleeping relatives gathered in his grandfather's dining room.

The occurrence of these illnesses in adults is extremely rare and children invariably outgrow them before adolescence. It is our strong opinion that these conditions should not be treated. I cannot overemphasize this point. Most treatments are ineffective and generally only make the child anxious for no good reason. In the end, patience is the only cure.

Drug Dependency: Insomniac Type

Now let us turn to an illness that is caused by the treatment. This is one of the somewhat paradoxical drug dependency sleep disorders. *The same pills people take to regulate their sleep cause profoundly disturbed sleep.* A large proportion of the patients we see in our clinic have drug-related sleep problems. Chief among these disorders is drug dependency insomnia caused by chronic ingestion of hypnotics.

Whenever an insomniac says he is taking sleeping pills, we assume that he has drug dependency insomnia. Current understanding of this syndrome is due largely to the efforts of one man, Dr. Anthony Kales, director of the Sleep Research and Treatment Facility at the Pennsylvania State University Medical School in Hershey, Pennsylvania. Many Americans will benefit from his findings.

Here is a typical case history of drug dependency insomnia: Mr. B. was studying for a civil service exam, the outcome of which would affect his entire future. He was terribly worried about the test and found it difficult to get to sleep at night. Feeling that the sleep loss was affecting his ability to study, he consulted his physician for the express purpose of getting "something to make me sleep." His doctor prescribed a moderate dose of barbiturate at bedtime, and Mr. B. found that this medication was very effective . . . for the first several nights. After about a week, he began having trouble sleeping again and decided to take two sleeping pills each night. Twice more the cycle was repeated, until on the night before the exam he was taking four times as many pills as his doctor had prescribed. The next night, with the pressure off, Mr. B. took no medication. He had terrific difficulty falling asleep, and when he did, his sleep was terribly disrupted for the rest of the night—he awoke often and had two disturbing nightmares. Mr. B. now decided that he had a serious case of insomnia, and returned to his sleeping pill habit. By the time he consulted our clinic several years later, he was taking approximately 1,000 mg sodium amytal every night, and his sleep was more disturbed than ever. Yet he had been perfectly normal before the transient stressful episode! Patients may go on for years and years—from one sleeping pill to another—never realizing that their troubles are *caused* by the pills.

Our recording of Mr. B.'s sleep while he was still addicted to barbiturates showed that his total sleep time was only about six hours a night with many awakenings and very little REM sleep or NREM Stages 3 and 4. The suppression of REM sleep by the medication was responsible for a large REM rebound when Mr. B. stopped taking the pills. The two nightmares reflected this rebound.

Almost every hypnotic compound will cause this syndrome when used chronically. These include sodium seconal, sodium amytal, sodium pentobarbital, barbital, sodium amobarbital and sodium secobarbital, glutethimide, methyprylon, and ethchlorvynol. Furthermore, in the absence of proof to the contrary, we have concluded that drug dependency will develop in any medication (including methaqualone and certain antihistamines) that shows a rapid development of tolerance to its sleep-inducing effects. The same principle applies to alcoholic beverages, popularly used as sleep medication.

Treatment of drug dependency insomnia is complete withdrawal of the sleep medication. A highly successful technique, introduced by Kales, involved the slow reduction of sleep medication at the rate of one therapeutic dose every week or ten days. Even under this very gradual withdrawal there is a possibility of nightmares. It is often quite difficult to treat this syndrome, primarily because some patients steadfastly maintain that any reduction of medication, however small, leaves them totally sleepless. In addition, they are often doubtful that forsaking their sleeping pills will cure them.

We must continually encourage these patients to remain in the withdrawal program. The greatest incentive we have to offer them is the fact that every patient who has completed withdrawal has greatly improved sleep and feels 100 percent better. Our patient, Mr. B., after struggling through the uncertainties of withdrawal, now serves as an example to others.

In hypnotic dependencies, it is extremely unwise to attempt acute ("cold turkey") withdrawal, particularly if the doses are high. It is always advisable to consult a doctor if withdrawal from any medication is contemplated. With barbiturates in particular, rapid withdrawal may lead to severe nightmares, and in some cases convulsive seizures.

Idiopathic Insomnia and Pseudo-Insomnia

If a patient complains of insomnia and *does not* take sleeping pills, we say that he has idiopathic insomnia. When we inaugurated the Stanford Sleep Disorders Clinic back in 1970, one of our very first and happiest decisions was to apply objective methods to the complaint of insomnia.

In spite of the effort and expense, we insisted that every patient have all-night sleep recordings to see exactly how much he or she slept. As the data piled up, we were more and more dumbfounded. Although every insomniac came to our clinic as their "last hope" in getting some respite from the tortures of sleeplessness, the severity of their complaint had *absolutely no relation* to the amount they slept in the laboratory!

Let's take a specific example. Mr. S. was a sixty-one-year-old single college professor. He had suffered chronically from insomnia since he was in college and would drag through his days sluggish and drowsy. He tried sleeping pills a few times, but quit because they didn't help. At the age of fifty-eight, he felt unable to continue teaching because of his insomnia and he officially retired.

Every patient who enters our clinic must keep a careful record of his sleep at home for at least one week. In addition, he must rate the way he feels on the Stanford Sleepiness Scale every fifteen minutes for one or two entire days. To make a presumptive diagnosis of idiopathic insomnia, we must see an average of six hours or less of sleep per day in the sleep diary, and signs of daytime sleepiness on the SSS. Mr. S. kept the diaries for two weeks and his average daily sleep time was three hours and fifty-nine minutes. It seemed clear that Mr. S. had a terrible sleep disturbance. We now had to define it. Accordingly, we required Mr. S. to sleep in the clinic laboratory for four consecutive nights. His average sleep time for the four nights was exactly eight hours and nine minutes! There was no possible doubt—one cannot question sleep spindles and slow waves in the EEG. Furthermore, we recorded two additional nights, giving Mr. S. an hypnotic dose of flurazepam at bedtime on each night. His sleep time on these two nights averaged seven hours and fifty-eight minutes.

Nearly half the patients who come to our clinic complaining that they cannot sleep are like Mr. S. The remainder actually appear to have a severe sleep disturbance. However, I wish to make one thing perfectly clear: There is absolutely no way of telling before the sleep recordings which patient will sleep and which one won't. Neither talking to them nor having them fill out diaries will tell them apart. Therefore, it is mandatory that every patient who seeks treatment for insomnia have all-night sleep recordings. Patients whose recordings show a normal amount of sleep *should not* be given any kind of sleeping pills. As we have seen, sleeping pills do nothing for these patients. At the present time, we call this condition pseudo-insomnia. We do not understand why pseudo-insomniacs feel they do not sleep at night, or why they feel sleepy and fatigued during the day. However, detailed knowledge about their sleep may save them years of crippling and useless dependency on sleeping pills. In the case of Mr. S., just knowing about his sleep was helpful. He subsequently wrote to us—"Now that I know that I get a normal amount of sleep, I don't fret and worry about sleeping. I seem to awaken less frequently during the night. I find that nowadays I am not particularly depressed. On the whole, I seem less tired too."

Those patients whose recordings *do* show disturbed sleep—who take hours to fall asleep, have frequent arousals during the night, awaken too early; who have, in short, very little sleep—can sometimes be helped with medication. However, the choice of medication is extremely important because, as we have noted, most sleeping pills make sleep worse. Extensive studies, particularly in Dr. Kales' laboratory, have shown one or two hypnotic compounds that seem to be relatively safe—dependency and tolerance do not immediately occur.

But what is the cause of all this suffering? Countless Americans cannot sleep well at night and cannot stay alert and awake through the day. However, sleep itself does not appear to explain the problem. Many totally normal uncomplaining people sleep only five hours a night, yet some insomniacs sleep more than eight. At the present time, we suspect that a disturbance in the basic mechanism of circadian oscillation may be at the root of these problems, but insomnia remains one of the greatest challenges to future sleep research.

Miles To Go

The foregoing descriptions should have conveyed some understanding of this new area of clinical medicine. Needless to say, our sleep disorders clinic is very busy. In addition to the conditions we have discussed, there are a host of others. Any complaint about sleep requires systematic and exhaustive evaluation.

Although these illnesses have always plagued mankind, they have remained until now cloaked in ignorance. There is no medical tradition for dealing with them, nor is there even a reasonably accurate folklore. If a middle-aged man experiences a severe pain in his chest, he will immediately think of his heart—even the most uninformed layman has some idea of underlying causation in the symptoms of heart disease. No physician would ever consider treating the symptom without further evaluation. No physician would just give a daily painkiller. Yet, this is pretty much the way most physicians approach sleep complaints. However, cardiology has more than one hundred years of tradition, while the sleep disorders have no tradition at all. Some complaints are treated by psychiatrists, some are treated by neurologists. Except for one or two places where expert help is available, no patient is properly evaluated by specialists trained in the sleep disorders. At this very moment, clinical sleep researchers are feverishly discovering and defining new illnesses of sleep and clarifying the old illnesses, while most physicians in the "real world" are still prescribing barbiturates and amphetamines for nearly everything. We have much work yet to do in both research *and* education. To paraphrase Robert Frost, we have miles to go before we sleep.

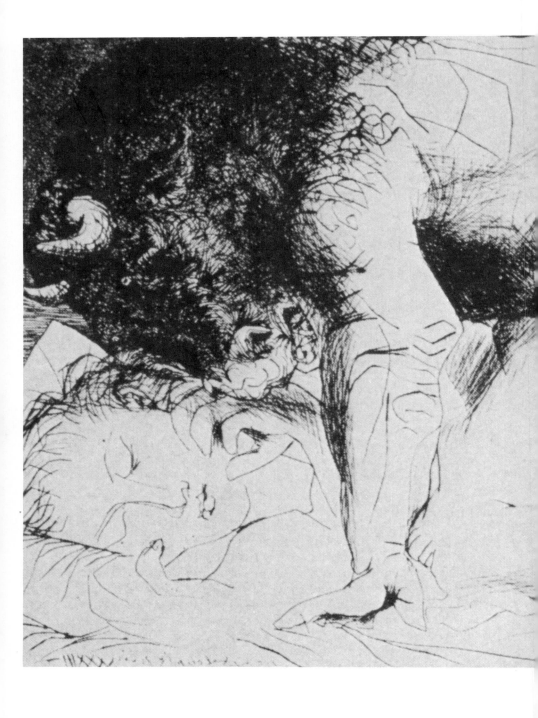

CHAPTER SIX

SLEEP DISTURBANCE AND MENTAL ILLNESS

HUGHLINGS JACKSON, THE GREAT NEUROLOGIST, said, "Find out about dreams and you will find out about insanity." The essence of dreaming is that we see, hear, smell, touch, and taste things that are not really there. If we were awake, the dream would be called an hallucination. Probably anyone who hallucinates is in some way insane, and all the more so if he believes in the reality of his hallucinations. We could say that dreaming is the prototypical hallucinatory experience. In other words, there is a possibility that the same process underlies both normal dreaming and abnormal hallucinations.

Because the dreams of REM sleep are "real" to the dreamer, and because the human memory must sort and process an incredible amount of information, it is not unusual for a person who is presumably sane to "remember" some dream detail as if it were fact. When this happens, we search the past and ask ourselves, "Did it really happen, or was it just a dream?" Such an occurrence may have been responsible for a disquieting experience I recently had.

At a basketball game in Stanford's Maples Pavilion, I happened to notice the team physician sitting on the bench and remembered that he had recently attended one of my lectures. After the game I intercepted the doctor on his way to the dressing room to tell him I was glad to know he was interested in sleep. In fact, I had been thinking about doing some research on the sleep habits of our Stanford athletes. I was astonished when I realized that the doctor didn't recognize me—and appalled when I learned that he had been in Chicago on the night of my lecture. Later, though I was quite disturbed, I concluded that a very plausible dream detail, the presence of a particular individual in the lecture room audience, had been temporarily preserved in my memory under the heading of fact. This experience, which may be nearly universal, illustrates the disruption of function that might occur if dream memories were frequently mistaken for waking reality.

It is no problem to label as "dreaming" any incongruity that has appeared in a dream. If I had dreamed of seeing a purple kangaroo in the lecture room, I would scarcely have remembered it as "fact." But our more prosaic dreams may overlap reality far more often than we know. Maybe a dream detail is being recalled when we say, "I *distinctly remember* putting that letter in my desk drawer, and now it isn't there!" or in an argument between two very positive antagonists, one of them shouting with obvious conviction, "I did not!" and the other declaring with equal conviction, "You did too! I *distinctly remember*." (Sanity depends upon a reliable memory. I don't think I could stand more than one such incongruity a day.)

A common notion about the relationship of sleep to mental health is that total sleep loss (both REM and NREM) deranges the mind and may result in some kind of breakdown. We have touched on this theme in Chapter One. When profound sleep disturbances are present, as they almost always are in the mentally ill, the patient's history often indicates that the sleep disturbance preceded the acute break with reality. Patients frequently say they would be all right if only they could get some sleep. Such observations raise the question whether sleep loss is one of the causes of mental illness or only one of the symptoms. At the very least, sleep is a sensitive barometer of psychic turbulence; it is virtually axiomatic that a disturbance of the mind will manifest itself in the sleeping state as well as as in the waking state.

Eugene Bliss of the Department of Psychiatry at the University of Utah has reported two cases of schizophrenia in which sleeplessness definitely preceded the acute break with reality. Although both of these patients were in their middle years, neither of them had experienced a previous schizophrenic episode. Each had a short-lived psychotic episode that responded rapidly to treatment. One of these histories is summarized as follows:

> The first patient was a forty-four-year-old woman who decompensated after the accidental death of her sixteen-year-old son. While driving the family car, he struck a cow and was

fatally injured. For the next twenty-seven hours he lingered in a coma and then died. During this time his mother stayed at his side. She cried, remained sleepless and complained of pains in the region of all her son's injuries. Thereafter, she became emotionally more controlled, but could not sleep. Her insomnia lasted almost three days, and at that time further evidences of irrationality were present. The next day, after close to ninety hours of sleep deprivation, self-recriminations and excruciating psychic distress, she became grossly psychotic. She railed against the atomic bomb, expressed religious delusions, refused to wear clothing, screamed and lapsed into an incomprehensible gibberish. She was taken to the hospital, and seven days later, after three electroshock treatments, reverted to normal behavior. Thereafter, she received two more electroshock treatments. Her behavior remained rational and she was discharged. Eight months later, at the time her son would have graduated from high school, a series of events reactivated her psychotic grief reaction. Again she became depressed, ruminative, and intensely miserable. She failed to sleep for three days, and relapsed into a psychotic state. She was rehospitalized, treated with chlorpromazine and perphenazine, and in six days, recovered. (From "Sleep in Schizophrenia and Depression—Studies of Sleep Loss in Man and Animals," in S. S. Kety, E. V. Evarts, and H. L. Williams (eds.), *Sleep and Altered States of Consciousness*; Baltimore: The Williams and Wilkins Co., 1967.)

We could add to these case presentations the story of Peter Tripp, the New York disc jockey mentioned earlier, as well as several others studied by Dr. West. But we must also remember Randy Gardner, who underwent 264 hours of continuous wakefulness without noticeable deterioration. Apparently, extended sleep loss does not always result in mental disorder. When it does, we tend to feel that the victim was predisposed to mental illness or was already schizophrenic or seriously depressed.

Another notion that arises from the almost superstitious awe in which some people hold their dreams is that dreams *are* madness and represent a kind of safety valve by which all of us can be quietly and safely mad every night of our lives. REM deprivation studies and studies of the depletion of certain neurotransmitters related to sleep have attempted to break down the barrier that prevents this nocturnal madness from entering into wakefulness.

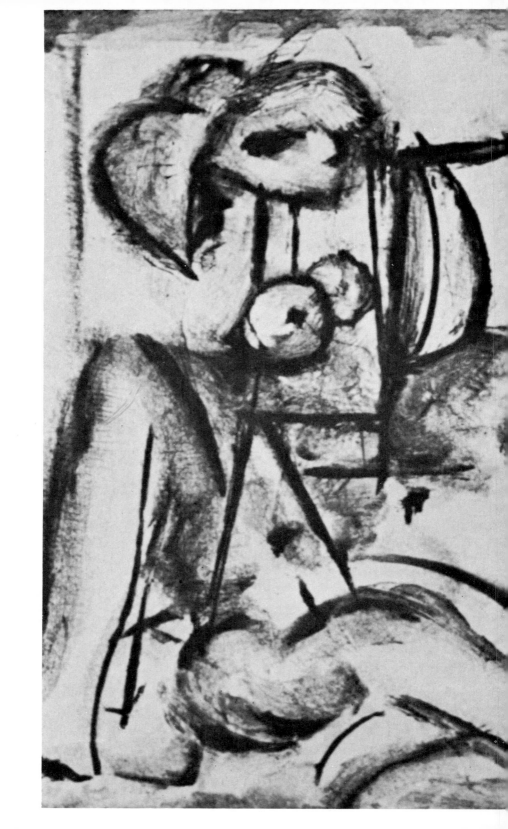

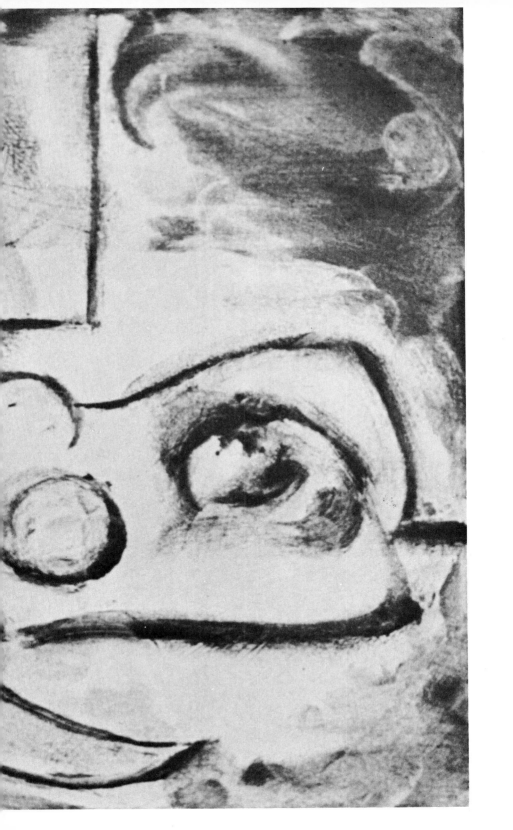

REM Deprivation

Because NREM sleep always precedes REM sleep, it is not possible to carry out selective deprivation of NREM sleep. It is possible, however, to deprive a subject selectively of REM sleep. One simply lets NREM sleep occur as usual, but interrupts each REM period at its onset. In this way, one can consider the effects of this state independently.

In 1959 Dr. Charles Fisher and I, working at the Mount Sinai Hospital in New York City, undertook the first study involving selective deprivation of REM sleep. In the back of our minds was some notion that if dreams were not allowed to occur during sleep, they might begin to occur during wakefulness. The subjects were two volunteers from the Columbia University Law School. Monitoring EEG and eye movements of both on a single machine, I attempted to prevent REM sleep by waking them whenever I saw the beginning of a REM period as indicated by the appearance of an eye movement burst. (Due to the lack of knowledge about motor inhibition at this time, I did not utilize the EMG, which has since become the most reliable indicator of the onset of REM sleep.)

Since this was the first time such a study had been attempted, I did not know precisely what to expect. I was therefore quite surprised when the number of arousals required to interrupt each REM period at its onset began to increase. By the third night I was trotting in and out of the subjects' bedrooms so fast that I could barely keep it up. My major aim, however, was to find out whether REM sleep would increase or decrease on the fourth night, the first recovery night.

After three very strenuous nights of monitoring, I approached this recovery night with considerable excitement. The subjects, who had been instructed to stay awake during the daytime, arrived at the lab around midnight; I hooked them up, put them to bed, and turned on the EEG machine. To my great dismay (ladies and gentlemen, this has happened more than once, but this is the only time I am going to moan about it) a horrible grinding from the EEG announced the fact that the paper drive system had broken down. Because it would have been impossible to replace this item at 1 a.m., I was forced to stop the experiment.

A few weeks later one of the subjects returned, and I conducted REM deprivation for five consecutive nights. REM onset awakenings increased from about seven the first night to more than fifteen on the fifth night. On the first recovery night, I was eager to see what would happen. The subject had gone through the first part of the NREM sleep cycle and was just beginning a REM period when a garbage truck stopped outside our tiny, two-room lab, and the clang and bang of garbage cans awakened the subject.

The subject went back to sleep, however, and fifteen minutes later he again entered a REM period. Past experience had indicated that the first REM period of the night would last about ten minutes. But this subject had a sixty-eight-minute REM period. His total REM time, which had averaged 16 percent on baseline nights, rose to 34 percent on this recovery night. We had discovered the "REM rebound," a dramatic increase in REM sleep that follows periods of REM deprivation.

Additional experiments with other subjects confirmed this result and seemed to suggest a specific need for REM sleep. In my report, published in *Science* in 1960, I noted that REM-deprived subjects showed anxiety, irritability, and difficulty in concentrating. I speculated that we might need a certain amount of REM sleep: REM deprivation seemed to lead to increased REM "pressure" which showed up as increasingly frequent onsets during the deprivation period and longer REM sleep in the recovery period. Implicit in this theory was the idea that if the deprivation were carried out for sufficiently lengthy durations, the dream-REM process would erupt into the waking state.

The idea had great appeal and launched an intensive investigation of REM deprivation in many laboratories—but a decade of research has failed to prove that substantial psychological ill effects result even from prolonged selective REM sleep deprivation. We have deprived human subjects of REM sleep for sixteen days, and cats for seventy consecutive days, without producing signs of serious psychological disruption.

While there have been signs of tremendous REM pressure—enormous increases and marked intensification of REM sleep in post-deprivation periods—there has been no sign that dreaming erupts into wakefulness under such stress. The barrier which prevents the REM sleep from spilling over into our waking hours is quite difficult to surmount.

Another approach to REM sleep deprivation resulted when Rechtschaffen and his group discovered that a certain drug, dextroamphetamine, would selectively suppress REM sleep. Thereafter Dexedrine was used in humans as an adjuvant to awakenings at the onset of REM periods. Other clinical investigations showed that alcohol suppresses REM sleep to some extent.

Several investigators, Dr. Milton Gross and his colleagues from the Downstate Medical Center in New York and Dr. Ramon Greenberg and his associates in Boston, have shown that delirium tremens, which follows acute withdrawal from alcohol in alcoholics, is associated with a remarkable alteration of sleep patterns. REM sleep approaches 100 percent of the total sleep time, and the hallucinations appear to be the breaking through of REM sleep in the waking psyche. As I mentioned earlier, barbiturates also suppress REM sleep, and their rapid withdrawal leads to REM sleep rebound and severe nightmares.

An especially interesting instance of this type of phenomenon was recently reported by Charles Fisher, who gave Nardil (a monoamine oxidase inhibitor) to a narcoleptic patient for the specific purpose of suppressing the REM sleep attacks. After several months of complete suppression, Fisher withdrew the Nardil, and the patient entered an almost continuous REM sleep interrupted by waking hallucinatory periods. Ian Oswald at the University of Edinburgh has seen similar experiences with the monoamine oxidase inhibitors.

Effects of Serotonin

Of course, REM sleep deprivation which is accomplished by chemical intervention could directly weaken the hypothetical barrier. As we try to identify the nature of the barrier, we have currently become very interested in a compound called serotonin. This compound is stored in the axon terminals of special nerve cells and serves as their neurotransmitter. In Chapter One I briefly alluded to the brilliant biochemical work of Jouvet and his colleagues at the University of Lyon, which suggested an important role for serotonin in the sleep mechanisms. They reported that the temporary inhibition of the synthesis of serotonin in the cat produces a fairly marked insomnia with a reduction of both REM and NREM sleep. Serotonin, which is normally produced in the brain, intestines, platelets, and many other organs, can be inhibited by the administration of a compound called parachlorophenylalanine (PCPA). We gave cats daily dosages of PCPA and found that, after a few days, the insomnia got better and the cats were able to sleep once more. But, dramatically, the phasic components of REM sleep, particularly the PGO spikes, began to emerge into the waking state. Thus, the more lasting effect of serotonin depletion was a disappearance of the barrier between REM sleep and wakefulness. The PCPA-treated cat could be described as a "waking dreamer," a description that has been applied also to the actively ill schizophrenic. We also found that we could not really produce REM sleep deprivation in the PCPA cat, probably because at least some parts of REM sleep were going on all the time. Although we were able to interrupt REM periods for several days, there was absolutely no REM rebound in the post-deprivation recovery period.

As the study of sleep delves further into the esoteric realms of biochemistry and neuropharmacology in laboratories around the world, sleep researchers dare to hope that a better understanding of dreaming and REM sleep will yield new ideas and new tools to investigate, and eventually to prevent, mental illness.

Sleep in Schizophrenics

The Stanford group has devoted a great deal of effort to the study of sleep in schizophrenic patients. Our earliest work involved all-night recording of undisturbed sleep in previously psychotic patients who were essentially normal at the time of recording. We found that their sleep patterns were also essentially normal. Our studies of selective REM sleep deprivation in schizophrenics were carried out in collaboration with Dr. Vincent Zarcone, Dr. George Gulevich, Dr. Terry Pivik, and Dr. Kazuo Azumi, who had come from Japan to work with us. We wanted to learn whether they had an abnormal response to deprivation as did the chronically treated PCPA cats reported above. We immediately stumbled upon the finding that schizophrenic subjects in remission appeared to show an excessive REM rebound after only two nights of REM deprivation.

In the course of these studies we also deprived subjects who were currently ill—hallucinating, delusional, showing bizarre behavior. These subjects appeared to have no rebound at all after two nights of REM deprivation. We were quite happy when Dr. Christopher Gillin and his colleagues at Saint Elizabeth's Hospital in Washington, D.C., reported a confirmation of the rebound failure in actively psychotic patients.

With an eye to the cat work mentioned earlier, we interpreted these findings as suggesting a possible serotonin defect in the currently ill schizophrenic patients. The defect would account for the intrusive hallucinations in the waking state and the rebound failure. As a logical next step, treatment of actively ill schizophrenics with a metabolic precursor of serotonin, 5-HTP (5-hydroxytryptophan) has been attempted by Dr. Richard Wyatt, also of Saint Elizabeth's Hospital. He has reported encouraging results.

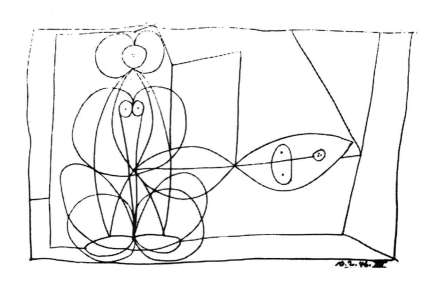

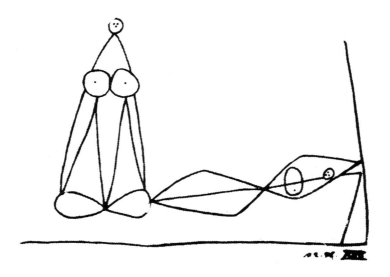

CHAPTER SEVEN

CREATIVITY DURING SLEEP

PERSONS WHO RESENT THE AMOUNT of time they must "waste" in sleep have attempted to make use of the nocturnal hours by combining sleep with productive mental activity. The most prevalent of these techniques is sleep-learning. Extravagant claims have been made for various commercially marketed sleep-teaching devices, nearly all of which utilize acoustical repetition of the material to be learned. In the hands of scientific investigators, however, such techniques have not been particularly successful.

A major difficulty has been the absence of an adequate demonstration that learning through these techniques actually takes place during sleep rather than during a succession of brief arousals occurring throughout the night. Charles W. Simon and William H. Emmons conducted experiments in which the addition of continuous EEG monitoring enabled them to present material only during sleep. Their results were completely negative.

It should be noted, however, that in one test these experimenters used complex questions and answers and presented each pair only once; in another test they used nonsense material. Some of the complex material might have been learned if it had been presented repeatedly. The nonsense material may have been disregarded because it had no relevance for the sleeping subjects. In view of these considerations, as well as recent demonstrations that both operant behavior and sensory discrimination can occur in humans during various levels of sleep, we may conclude that the possibility of certain kinds of learning (perhaps low-efficiency learning) during sleep has not been conclusively eliminated.

An accumulation of anecdotal evidence supports the possibility that sleeping time can be used, though not deliberately, for mental activities usually confined to the waking state. Two examples are problem solving and artistic creation. Most occurrences of such high-level mental performance during sleep have been attributed to dreams. Since we now know that dreaming is an intrinsic part of sleeping and occupies a specific and substantial portion of every night's sleep, we may assume that the opportunity for "creative dreaming" is potentially available to everyone.

Artistic Creations

Probably the most famous example of creative dreaming is the poem "Kubla Khan" by Samuel Taylor Coleridge, which John Livingston Lowes has called "one of the most remarkable poems in the English language." In 1816 Coleridge published an account of its genesis. He had retired to a lonely farmhouse in Devonshire for reasons of ill health. Laudanum (tincture of opium) had been prescribed for a "slight indisposition," and its effects caused him to fall asleep in his chair while he was reading the following lines from "Purchas' Pilgrimage": "Here the Khan Kubla commanded a palace to be built, and a stately garden thereunto. And thus ten miles of fertile ground were enclosed with a wall."

Coleridge said that he slept soundly for more than an hour, during which time he composed two or three hundred lines in a dream. Upon awakening, he took his pen, ink, and paper and instantly and eagerly wrote down the lines that have been preserved. He was unfortunately interrupted by a visitor who detained him for more than an hour. When he was able to return to the poem, some eight or ten scattered lines and a few sensory impressions were all that remained in his memory. "All the rest had passed away like the images on the surface of a stream into which a stone has been cast."

In his thoughtful study of "Kubla Khan" and "The Ancient Mariner," *The Road to Xanadu*, Lowes has shown that Coleridge, in his reading and notes made therefrom, had already encountered many of the individual ideas or images expressed in these poems; but the creation of "Kubla Khan" certainly occurred during sleep.

Coleridge was known to be an habitual user of laudanum. Little is known about the nature of sleep induced by narcotics, but evidence from sleep laboratories indicates that some measures of sleep remain within normal limits following habituation, and that the dreaming phase is slightly enhanced. Coleridge published a quatrain that came to him in sleep when he was not under the influence of laudanum:

> Here lies at length poor Col' and with screaming,
> Who died, as he had always lived, a dreaming:
> Shot dead, while sleeping, by the gout within,
> Alone, and all unknown, at E'nbro' in an Inn.

Another poem, "The Phoenix," was composed during sleep by A. C. Benson, the English essayist. Benson wrote, "I dreamt the whole poem in a dream, and wrote it down in the middle of the night on a scrap of paper by my bedside. I have never had a similar experience before or since. I can really offer no explanation either of the idea of the poem or its interpretation. It came to me so apparently without any definite volition of my own that I don't profess to understand or be able to interpret the symbolism."

> By feathers green, across Casbeen,
>   The pilgrims track the Phoenix flown,
> By gems he strewed in waste and wood
>   And jewelled plumes at random thrown.
>
> Till wandering far, by moon and star,
>   They stand beside the fruitful pyre,
> Whence breaking bright with sanguine light,
>   The impulsive bird forgets his sire.
>
> Those ashes shine like ruby wine,
>   Like bag of Tyrian murex spilt;
> The claw, the jowl of the flying fowl
>   Are with the glorious anguish gilt.
>
> So rare the light, so rich the sight,
>   Those pilgrim men, on profit bent,
> Drop hands and eyes and merchandise,
>   And are with gazing most content.

In his book, *The Unconscious*, Morton Prince reproduced a long poem and an account of its dream derivation. Apparently Prince awoke from the dream and wrote a description of it more or less unconsciously in poetic form. Robert Louis Stevenson, in his autobiography, *Across the Plains*, describes some of his dream life and credits his dreams for the plots of many of his stories, most notably *Doctor Jekyll and Mister Hyde*. The inspiration for the famous *Devil's Trill Sonata* came to Tartini in a dream in which he saw and heard the devil take up a violin and play the music that Tartini wrote down upon awakening.

The foregoing examples have been documented from autobiographical sources. There are literally hundreds of apparently apocryphal stories published without documentation. In *The Twilight Zone of Dreams*, André Sonnet credits dreaming for nearly every artistic and technological achievement accomplished by our race. He stated, for example, that the planetary model of the atom had come to Nobel Prize winner Niels Bohr in a dream. I wrote Bohr to obtain verification. He responded, somewhat bluntly, that he had never had a useful dream as far as he knew; and furthermore, it was Lord Rutherford who had conceived the model of orbiting electrons.

Problem Solving

A dream *was* the inspiration for "the most brilliant piece of prediction to be found in the whole range of organic chemistry," the structure of the benzene ring. After many years of fruitless effort to solve the structural riddle of the benzene molecule (C_6H_6), Friedrich August Kekulé, a German chemist, had a dream in which he saw six snakes biting each other's tails and whirling around in a circle. When he awoke, he interpreted the six snakes as a hexagon and immediately recognized the elusive structure of benzene. Another remarkable dream has been recorded by Hermann Hilprecht, a professor of Assyrian, in which a priest came to him and told him the true translation of the Stone of Nebuchadnezzar, which later proved to be correct. Also originated in a dream was the frog heart experiment, the results of which became the foundation of the theory of chemical transmission of nerve impulses and earned a Nobel Prize for the author, Otto Loewi.

Another Nobel Prize winner, Albert Szent-Gyorgyi, stated, "My work is not finished when I leave my workbench in the afternoon. I go on thinking about my problems all the time, and my brain must continue to think about them when I sleep because I wake up, sometimes in the middle of the night, with answers to questions that have been puzzling me."

It is likely that artistic creation and problem solving occur in dreams more often than the documentation suggests. An intense waking preoccupation appears to be an important factor, and this preoccupation depends, to some extent, upon the significance of the problem and the motivation of the individual seeking a solution. The problems of Kekulé, Otto Loewi, and Hilprecht had occupied their energies for many years.

The creative and problem-solving functions of dreams have been almost totally ignored by scientific investigators. The subject was approached as early as 1892 by Charles M. Child, who gathered some statistics. In a questionnaire distributed to 151 male and forty-nine female college students, he asked: "During sleep have you ever pursued a logically connected train of thought upon some topic or problem in which you have reached some conclusion, and the steps and conclusion of which you remembered upon awakening?" Of 186 students who responded to this question, sixty-two or 33.3 percent answered in the affirmative. Some of the examples given were a chess game played in a dream, an algebra problem solved, a bookkeeping error found, and a translation of Virgil accomplished.

At Stanford we explored the phenomenon of problem solving in dreams through a series of problem-solving experiments involving 500 undergraduate students in three consecutive class meetings. Each student was given a copy of a problem and an accompanying questionnaire and instructed not to look at the problem until fifteen minutes before he went to bed that night. Before going to bed the student was to spend exactly fifteen minutes in an attempt to solve the problem. In the morning he was supposed to write on the questionnaire any dream recalled from the previous night. If the problem had not been solved, the student was supposed to work on it for another fifteen minutes in the morning. The student's solution to the problem was entered on the questionnaire, which was then returned to the instructor to be scored by several volunteers who were looking for solutions that could be attributed to dreams. The students were instructed not to discuss the problem among themselves until the next class meeting. Here are the three problems and their solutions:

Problem 1: The letters O, T, T, F, F . . . form the beginning of an infinite sequence. Find a simple rule for determining any or all successive letters. According to your rule, what would be the next two letters of the sequence?

Solution 1: The next two letters in the sequence are S, S. The letters represent the first letters used in spelling out the numerical sequence, "One, Two, Three, Four, Five, Six, Seven, etc."

Problem 2: Consider the letters H, I, J, K, L, M, N, O. The solution to this problem is one word. What is this word?

Solution 2: The solution is the word "water" derived from the chemical formula H_2O or H-to-O as given in the problem.

Problem 3: The numbers 8, 5, 4, 9, 1, 7, 6, 3, 2 form a sequence. How are these numbers ordered?

Solution 3: The numbers, if spelled out, are ordered alphabetically.

The total response represented 1,148 attempts at problem solving. Using a rather intricate scoring system, we judged that eighty-seven dreams were related to the problem, fifty-three directly and thirty-four indirectly. If a solution was presented in the dream, the judges scored it as correct or incorrect, whether or not the subject recognized it as such. The correct solution appeared only nine times—all in the first experiment. On two of these occasions, however, the solution that appeared in the dream had already been obtained by the subject during the fifteen minutes before bed. Of the 1,148 attempts, therefore, the problem was solved in a dream on only seven occasions.

The following dream report contained one of these solutions:

"I was standing in an art gallery looking at the paintings on the wall. As I walked down the hall, I began to count the paintings— one, two, three, four, five. But as I came to the sixth and seventh, the paintings had been ripped from their frames! I stared at the empty frames with a peculiar feeling that some mystery was about to be solved. Suddenly I realized that the sixth and seventh spaces were the solution to the problem!"

In the second experiment there were twelve dreams classified as "mode of expression dreams" in which the answer, "water," was referred to either directly or indirectly. An example of the mode of expression dream was submitted by a nineteen-year-old male student— who solved the problem incorrectly with the word "alphabet." His dream recall was as follows:

"I had several dreams, all of which had *water* in them somewhere. In one dream I was hunting for sharks. In another I was riding waves at the ocean. In another I was confronted by a barracuda while skin diving. In another dream it was raining quite heavily. In another I was sailing into the wind." (This student probably did not recognize the word "water" as the correct solution because he had already solved the problem to his own satisfaction.)

While this experiment had several drawbacks in terms of design and controls, we feel that it may give a valid indication of the possibility, albeit rarely evidenced, of problem solving during sleep. The design of the experiment had several obvious shortcomings. Most of the anecdotal incidents of problem solving in dreams involved men who had been struggling with a particular problem for many years; our students had worked on the problem for only fifteen minutes. Even the most diligent and conscientious student had little incentive to obtain a solution, and this difficulty was probably more significant with the second and third experiments as the novelty decreased. In any experiment dealing with dreams, there is no assurance that the reported dreams are actually experienced by the subjects. We could not prevent the students from studying the problem prematurely or discussing it among themselves. We are convinced, however, that the dream solutions obtained in this experiment were valid examples of problem solving.

A contemporary example of problem solving in dreams was described in the *San Francisco Chronicle* of June 27, 1964. Jack Nicklaus, the professional golfer, had slumped badly after winning a number of championships. After suddenly regaining his championship form, he told a newspaper reporter: "I've been trying everything to find out what has been wrong. It was getting to the place where I figured a 76 was a pretty good round. But last Wednesday night I had a dream and it was about my golf swing. I was hitting them pretty good in the dream and all at once I realized I wasn't holding the club the way I've actually been holding it lately. I've been having trouble collapsing my right arm taking the club head away from the ball, but I was doing it perfectly in my sleep. So when I came to the course yesterday morning, I tried it the way I did in my dream and it worked. I shot a 68 yesterday and a 65 today and believe me it's a lot more fun this way. I feel kind of foolish admitting it, but it really happened in a dream. All I had to do was change my grip just a little."

In the minds of most human beings, sleep is too commonplace to deserve careful consideration, and dreams are too "foolish" to suggest a logical course of action that might be carried out in the waking state. The intricate clockwork that regulates the alternating phases of our daily life cycle is far more delicate than many of us realize. Without a second thought we make havoc of our normal cyclic variations by staying up too late too often, taking drugs to induce sleep and more drugs to wake up, drinking enormous quantities of coffee or tea, taking too many transoceanic flights, or consuming quantities of alcohol. And while we treat our sleep with indifference, we treat our dreams with contempt.

We cannot eliminate the possibility that all of us are presented solutions to our problems quite regularly in our dreams. Perhaps only the most perceptive dreamers possess the ability to recognize a solution that is presented in a disguised or symbolic fashion. Most of us, most of the time, are like the student who failed to recognize the word "water" as the solution to his problem even though he was deluged by water in his dreams! One can easily imagine Kekulé shrugging as he awakened from the dream of the six circling snakes: "What nonsense! I must forget about snakes and concentrate on chemistry."

I know of another, perhaps potentially more meaningful, way in which dreams may have a problem-solving function. Some years ago I was a heavy cigarette smoker—up to two packs a day. Then one night I had an exceptionally vivid and realistic dream in which I had inoperable cancer of the lung. I remember as though it were yesterday looking at the ominous shadow in my chest X-ray and realizing that the entire right lung was infiltrated. The subsequent physical examination in which a colleague detected widespread metastases in my axiliary and inguinal lymph nodes was equally vivid. Finally, I experienced the incredible anguish of knowing my life was soon to end, that I would never see my children grow up, and that none of this would have happened if I had quit cigarettes when I first learned of their carcinogenic potential. I will never forget the surprise, joy, and exquisite relief of waking up. I felt I was reborn. Needless to say, the experience was sufficient to induce an immediate cessation of my cigarette habit. This dream had both anticipated the problem, and had solved it in a way that may be a dream's unique privilege.

Only the dream can allow us to experience a future alternative as if it were real, and thereby to provide a supremely enlightened motivation to act upon this knowledge.

As a parting salute, I offer my all-time favorite quotation about dreaming, courtesy of Havelock Ellis—one that says it all: "Dreams are real while they last. Can we say more of life?"

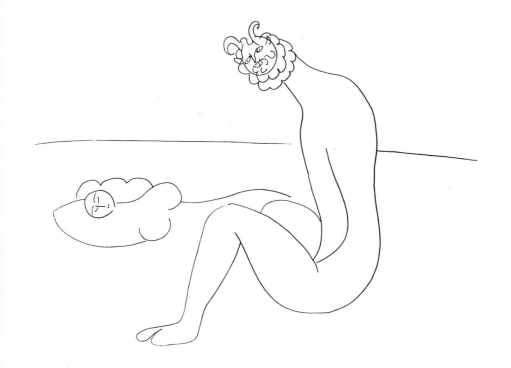

APPENDIXES

**FIGURES
GLOSSARY
READER'S GUIDE**

A

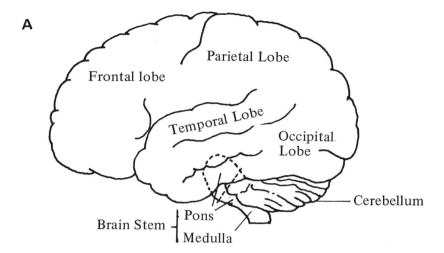

Frontal lobe

Parietal Lobe

Temporal Lobe

Occipital Lobe

Cerebellum

Brain Stem — Pons

Medulla

B

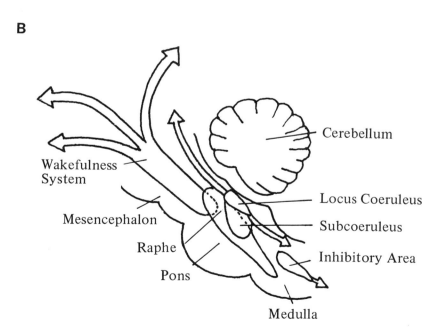

Cerebellum

Wakefulness System

Locus Coeruleus

Subcoeruleus

Mesencephalon

Inhibitory Area

Raphe

Pons

Medulla

Figure 1: The Brain Stem and the Sleep-Wakefulness Systems

A. In this drawing of the brain you can see that the brain stem, which houses the sleep mechanisms, is quite small in comparison with the great lobes of convoluted neocortex. The divisions of the brain stem from spinal cord up are *medulla oblongata, pons, mesencephalon,* and *diencephalon.* The pons and mesencephalon are the more crucial areas in terms of sleep and wakefulness. Structurally, the brain stem is a cylinder of neural tissue connecting the spinal cord to the rest of the brain. Strategically, this is obviously the best place from which to exert control.

B. This longitudinal view of the brain stem shows the cell bodies of neurons in the various "control" systems. These cells exert their control by means of tiny filaments called *axons* which project to many areas of the brain. After the axon divides, subdivides, re-subdivides, etc., one of these "control" centers may "drive" a population of more than 100,000 cells in the neocortical mantle and other areas of the brain. The cells that seem important in initiating and maintaining wakefulness are located mainly in the mesencephalon. Cells that probably play a role in NREM sleep are located in the *Raphe nuclei,* mainly in the pons and posterior mesencephalon. The *nucleus locus coeruleus* (it means blue plane) and the *nucleus subcoeruleus* seem to coordinate REM sleep. The medullary inhibitory area is thought to be the common pathway for all motor inhibition. It must be massively activated during REM sleep and cataplexy.

C. A cross section of the brain stem at the pons level shows the raphe, or serotonergic neurons, right in the midline of the brain stem. The locus coeruleus (REM?) cells are more lateral. The mesencephalic wakefulness neurons (not shown) are also more lateral in their distribution. While I don't want to undermine the reader's confidence, I must mention that the schema depicted, although strongly supported by laboratory experiments, is nonetheless hypothetical. Providing proof that any area of the brain has a specific function is always difficult. In a relatively inaccessible area like the brain stem, it's nearly impossible.

C

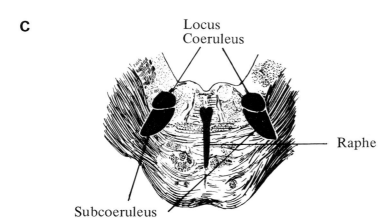

Locus
Coeruleus

Raphe

Subcoeruleus

Figure 2: Circadian Rhythm in Sleep and Wakefulness

2A. This day-by-day plot of a single individual's sleep and wakefulness illustrates one aspect of the circadian oscillation. The solid lines indicate sleep, the dotted lines indicate wakefulness, and the symbol ▲ indicates the low point of the body temperature during each successive twenty-four-hour period. The upper nine periods show sleep and wakefulness during a nine-day interval in a normal environment where we are exposed to alternating sunlight and darkness, warmth and coldness, noise and quiet. These and many other factors in our environment that change rhythmically because of the earth's rotation "entrain" our endogenous circadian oscillation to a periodicity of exactly twenty-four hours. This is why we tend to go to bed and get up about the same time each day. Days four and five represent a typical weekend sleep pattern, with a later bedtime and arising time on two consecutive days. However, on the mornings after the later bedtimes it is difficult to continue sleeping until eight hours of sleep have been accumulated because the entrained circadian oscillation continues without interruption and this means we are trying to sleep when the cycle is on the upswing. Note that the lowest body temperature occurs toward the end of sleep each night.

The middle section of the plot is very important. It illustrates what would happen if the individual were placed in a situation isolated from the normal environment and all the influences of the earth's rotation. In such an environment, temperature, noise levels, etc., would be constant. He would control the light himself, prepare his own meals when he was hungry, etc. There would be no clues (clocks, etc.) to tell him what time it was. Such an environment would have to be a cave or bunker deep underground.

The first important point is that the circadian oscillation in bodily functions would continue. It is innate, internal, built into the organism, and does not need to be "driven" from outside. The second important point is that the oscillation would no longer be exactly twenty-four hours. In an isolated environment, the individual would "free run." The latter term applies when the circadian rhythm is no longer entrained to twenty-four hours by environmental influences, but rather is oscillating at its own natural periodicity. The individual does things when he "feels like it." What is remarkable is that in such a case, the sleep-wakefulness rhythm of the body shows a periodicity that is close to twenty-four hours. In the case we have illustrated, the internal clock of the individual has a natural rhythm of exactly twenty-five hours. Thus, as he goes to bed when he becomes sleepy, his sleep starts about one hour later each night. During twenty-four days in isolation he drifts all the way around the clock until he is going to sleep at midnight again. Although it would not be exactly twenty-five hours, the natural oscillation of most people would probably be from about twenty-four and a half hours to twenty-five and a half hours. This is why the term circadian—circa, around, close to, and dies, day—is so appropriate to describe these natural oscillations. When our subject was "free running," the body temperature rhythm changed its phase relationship to sleep-wakefulness. Instead of reaching its low point toward the end of sleep, the low point occurred at the beginning of the sleep period. This change in the phase relationship is evidence that body temperature is an independent oscillator.

The lower section of the figure illustrates the course of events when the individual leaves isolation and becomes re-entrained to a twenty-four-hour day. Such re-entrainment is obviously easier when he has drifted all the way around the clock, than if he emerged from isolation when he was going to bed at around noon. At any rate, as before the isolation experiment, the lights are turned off at midnight and turned on around 8 a.m. Meals are served at a certain time each day. Note that the bedtime becomes stable at around midnight and the low point of body temperature moves back toward the end of the sleep period.

Most humans, as we have indicated, have a natural periodicity of approximately twenty-five hours, which is easily entrained to the twenty-four-hour day. However, we postulate that in insomniacs and other sleep-disordered patients, something may be wrong with either the entrainment mechanism or the innate oscillation so that their bodies cannot oscillate in synchrony with their environment.

Circadian Oscillation of Vigilance States in Natural, "Free Running," and Entrained Situations

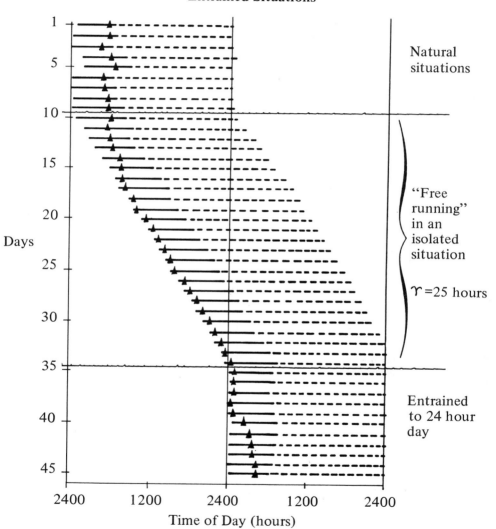

Days

Time of Day (hours)

Natural situations

"Free running" in an isolated situation

Υ =25 hours

Entrained to 24 hour day

2B. This is a somewhat idealized graph of a person's body temperature, showing its more or less sinusoidal fluctuation throughout the day and night. Note that the maximum temperature occurs during the day and the minimum at night. This is a very good example of the circadian oscillation that is present in nearly all bodily functions. In the old days, people thought that the low nocturnal body temperature was a passive consequence of the general absence of muscle activity during sleep. However, as we have shown in the figure, the daily temperature cycle continues even if we do not sleep. The intrinsic circadian rhythms of bodily functions are not dependent upon the daily alternation of sleep-wakefulness. Rather, the circadian fluctuations influence the tendency to sleep or remain awake. The jet lag syndrome suffered by world travelers clearly illustrates this principle. Such travelers must change their clocks but cannot immediately change the smooth flow of their circadian rhythms, and, therefore, the trough of the oscillation occurs during the day, which makes them very drowsy, and the peak occurs at night, which makes their sleep fitful and restless.

Circadian Oscillation of Body Temperature

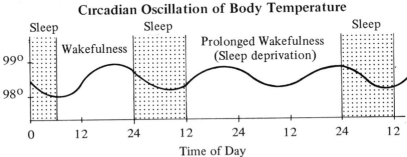

Time of Day

Figure 3: Hookup

This is a drawing of the "standard" setup for studying sleep in the laboratory. It shows the points on the scalp and face where electrodes are placed for the polygraphic sleep recording. These electrodes are small silver discs that are slightly cupped to hold a minute amount of electrode jelly. They are held in place by small pieces of sticky plastic tape. The procedure is entirely without pain or discomfort.

Every subject or patient whose sleep is studied in the laboratory will have this standard hookup. In addition, there may be additional attachments for measuring other functions such as breathing, heartbeat, body temperature, penile tumescence, and so on. Even when they sometimes have enough attachments to look like a Christmas tree, subjects have no difficulty sleeping.

The wires from the scalp and facial electrodes (and other attachments if they are present) are gathered into a pony tail at the back of the head and each wire is plugged into the jack box on the headboard. A cable leads from the jack box to the polygraph, which amplifies the brain wave, eye movement, and muscle potentials and writes them out on the moving chart paper. The speed at which the paper moves obviously makes a difference in the appearance of the EEG undulations. The standard speed for sleep recordings is 10 millimeters per second, which means that an average night of sleep requires about one thousand feet of chart paper. The polygraph and other recording apparatus is always housed in a separate room so as not to disturb the sleeper.

The tracings you see in the figure illustrate the write-out as it would be seen in an actual recording. They also show why these three measures (EEG, EOG, EMG) are always recorded. In this example, we see a transition from NREM sleep to REM sleep. Such a transition can be said to have occurred only when the muscle activity (EMG) ceases, brain waves (EEG) are more active, and eye movement potentials (EOG) are seen. In the absence of one of these three important criteria, we cannot be sure what kind of sleep is actually present. Note that the eye movement tracings move up and down in opposition to one another. This does not mean that the eyes are looking in opposite directions, but indicates, rather, that the two eyes are looking in the same direction. The latter is called binocular synchrony. The reason for the opposition of the EOG potentials is that the polarity at an electrode depends upon whether the eyes roll toward or away from it. Thus, if the subject looks to the right, the electrode on the right becomes positive, the electrode on the left becomes negative, and the pens move in opposite directions. When he looks to the left, the polarity is reversed.

We must re-emphasize that the subject is perfectly comfortable. The pony tail allows plenty of room to roll around or even sit up. The moderate noise of the polygraph and other machinery of the sleep laboratory does not penetrate into the soundproof bedroom. Accordingly, the subject sleeps peacefully through the night, virtually oblivious to the fact that every second of his sleep is being carefully analyzed.

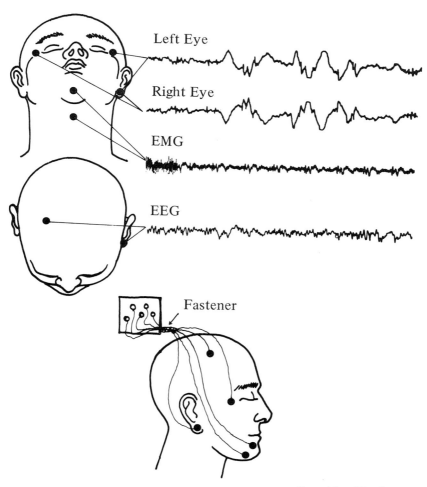

Left Eye

Right Eye

EMG

EEG

Fastener

Awake

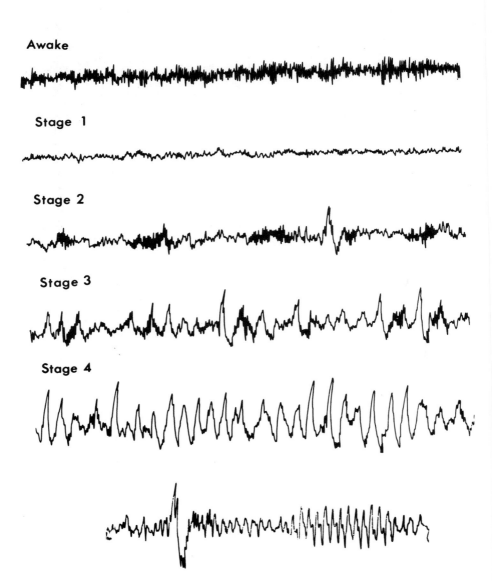

Stage 1

Stage 2

Stage 3

Stage 4

Figure 4: Stages of Sleep

This figure shows sample EEG tracings which illustrate the typical patterns seen in wakefulness, the four NREM EEG stages, and REM sleep. The top five lines represent thirty seconds of brain wave recording while the bottom line is eight seconds. All were recorded at the standard chart speed of 10 millimeters per second. A 10-millimeter deflection of the recording pen up or down represents a potential change in the brain of about 50 millionths of a volt (microvolts). The first line shows the normal brain wave pattern of relaxed wakefulness. Note the presence of an almost continuous, relatively fast sinusoidal rhythm. This is the well-known alpha rhythm whose fluctuations are characteristically close to 10 cycles per second. As you can see, no rhythmic wave forms stand out in the EEG patterns of NREM Stage 1. The patterns are typically of low amplitude and relatively fast mixed frequencies. In NREM Stage 2, the sleep spindles and K complexes (one is seen in the last third of the tracing) are characteristic features of the EEG. The sleep spindle is a rhythmic burst of 12-14 cps waves that wax and wane dramatically over an interval of one or two seconds. As in this example, the background EEG activity of Stage 2 is of very low amplitude against which the sleep spindles and K complexes stand out very clearly. These two complex EEG wave forms appear *only* during NREM sleep. They never appear in wakefulness, and if they occasionally appear in what seems to be a period of REM sleep, it usually signals a brief interruption of the REM period. Sleep spindles may also be seen in NREM Stage 3. However, the determinant of this stage is the appearance of high amplitude, slow waves. These are called delta waves and are rhythmic oscillations at a rate of about one-half to two per second. When more than one-half of the tracing contains delta waves that exceed seventy-five microvolts in amplitude, it is called Stage 4. Thus, Stage 3 is essentially an intermediate stage between 2 and 4.

The last tracing shows the EEG transition from NREM Stage 2 to REM sleep. In the early portion of the tracing, a well-defined K complex is very obvious, indicating that it is Stage 2 sleep. The EEG patterns in the middle of the tracing are transitional. REM sleep is evidenced by the characteristic and unique wave forms called "saw-tooth waves" in the last few seconds of the sample. If eye movements and muscle activity were recorded simultaneously with these saw-tooth waves, we would expect to see that EMG activity was suppressed and eye movements were present. If the EMG were not suppressed, we could not call it REM sleep in spite of the presence of saw-tooth waves.

Figure 5: Course of Events

This figure is a plot of REM sleep, NREM sleep, and the four stages of NREM sleep over the course of one entire night of sleep. Although it is a "real" night from one particular subject, it is also a representative night. In other words, with a few minor changes, most nights of most people would show the identical sequence of events. The time spent in NREM sleep is lightly shaded and the time spent in REM sleep is shown in black. NREM sleep always is the first to occur at the beginning of the night. It is abnormal to go from daytime wakefulness directly into REM sleep. The first period of NREM sleep usually lasts about an hour and then gives way to the first period of REM sleep. From the onset of sleep to the end of the first REM period is the first *sleep cycle*. From the end of the first REM period to the end of the second REM period is the second sleep cycle, and so on. Thus, the cyclic alternation of NREM and REM sleep is what constitutes the basic sleep cycle that is often referred to in the literature. The average periodicity of this cycle is ninety minutes, although individual cycles may show considerable variation in length. The first sleep cycle is usually somewhat short, about seventy to eighty minutes; the second and third are usually longer than average, 100 to 110 minutes; later cycles tend to be a little shorter.

As you can see, Stages 3 and 4 dominate the NREM periods in the first part of the night, but are completely absent during the later cycles. Thus, we say that sleep is deepest in the first third of the night because we feel that it is harder to wake people up from Stage 4 sleep. The amount of Stage 2 sleep becomes progressively greater as the night wears on until it completely occupies the NREM periods toward the end of the night. The first REM period is usually relatively short, five to ten minutes, but tends to lengthen in successive cycles. Here again, individual REM periods show great variability in length, although the overall average is about twenty-two minutes. Toward the end of the night, very brief periods of wakefulness may interrupt sleep. This happens to each of us nearly every night although we may never even notice the little awakenings. In this example of an entire night, the brief periods of wakefulness were in NREM sleep, but short awakenings often occur in REM sleep as well.

Sequences of States and Stages of Sleep on a Typical Night

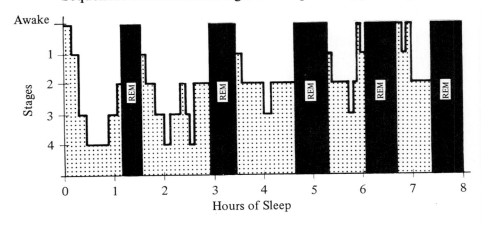

Figure 6: Mammoth Cave, Kentucky, 1938

Nathaniel Kleitman and B. H. Richardson emerge from Mammoth Cave after thirty-two days in a damp and chilly subterranean chamber. During this time they lived in near total isolation from the outside world, attempting to adjust to a twenty-eight-hour daily schedule of nineteen wakeful hours and nine hours in bed. As they were greeted by the local dignitaries, I am sure that they were thinking more of a hot bath and a warm bed than of the ceremony.

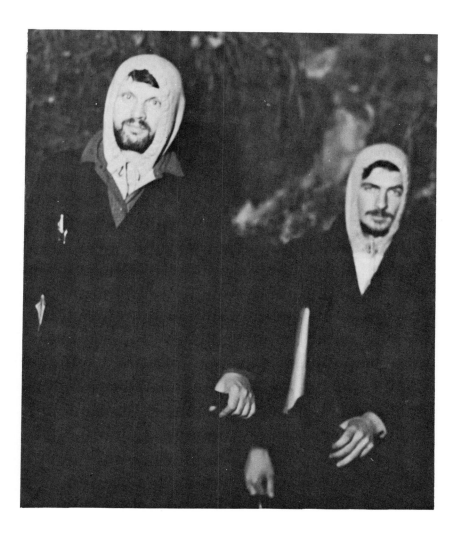

Figure 7: Compilation of Results From Dream Recall Studies in REM and NREM Sleep

Study	Number of Subjects	Number of Subject Nights	Number of REM Period Awakenings		Number of NREM Sleep Awakenings	
			Dream Recall	No Dream Recall	Dream Recall	No Dream Recall
University of Chicago Sleep Lab—1955 (Eugene Aserinsky and Nathaniel Kleitman)	10	14	20	7	4	19
University of Chicago Sleep Lab—1955 (William Dement)	10	18	45	6	0	19
University of Chicago Sleep Lab—1957 (William Dement and Nathaniel Kleitman)	9	61	152	39	11	149
University of New York Sleep Lab, Downstate Medical Center—1959 (Donald Goodenough et al.)	16	48	63	28	34	65
University of Lyon, France, Sleep Lab—1960 (Michel Jouvet, J. Dechaume, and François Michel)	4	15	12	8	1	29
National Institute of Mental Health Sleep Lab—1960 (Frederick Snyder)	30	96	291	66	12	77
University of Chicago Sleep Lab (2nd Generation)—1960 (Edward Wolpert)	8	20	27	10	5	16
University of Chicago Sleep Lab (2nd Generation)—1958 (Edward Wolpert and Harry Trosman)	10	51	131	46	0	37
TOTALS:	97	323	771	210	67	411
PERCENTAGES:			78.6	21.4	14.0	86.0

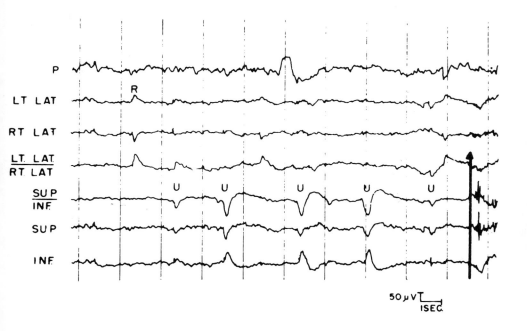

P

LT LAT

RT LAT

LT LAT
RT LAT

SUP
INF

SUP

INF

50 μV
1 SEC.

Figure 8: Eye Movements

These recordings were taken from REM periods just before the subjects were awakened for the purpose of giving a detailed account of the dream events immediately preceding the arousing buzzer. They will illustrate the remarkable correspondence between eye movement sequences and events in the dream that we sometimes obtain.

In the above sample, the top line is the EEG tracing and all others are eye movements. For this study, the eye movements were recorded from several different locations including the sides of the eyes (for recording leftward and rightward eye movements) and above and below the eyes (for recording upward and downward movements). The direction of eye movements is indicated on the figure: R—eyes have moved to the right; and U—eyes have moved upward. This figure is the actual recording made on the subject mentioned in the discussion of the scanning hypothesis. As you can see, the eye movements shown here are exactly as the interrogator, Dr. Roffwarg, predicted from the subject's dream report.

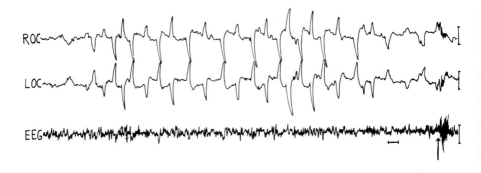

ROC

LOC

EEG

The eye movements in the above figure were recorded from the outside corner of the left eye or LOC (left outer canthus) and from the outside corner of the right eye or ROC (right outer canthus). When the subject looks to the right, the ROC pen moves down and the LOC pen moves up; the opposite takes place when he looks to the left. The sequence of eye movements in this REM period sample is truly amazing. It consisted of no less than twenty-six regularly spaced to-and-fro horizontal movements with no vertical components whatsoever. Such a totally non-random and distinctively patterned eye movement sequence is quite a rare occurrence. When such a sequence does occur, it is always an excellent opportunity to examine the relationship between dream content and direction of eye movements. In this example, the subject was awakened (arrow) immediately following the horizontal eye movements and asked to report his dream. He stated that he had been watching a ping pong game between two friends. In the dream, he had stood at the side of the ping pong table so that he had to look from side to side to watch the ball. He also reported that he had been watching a rather long volley just before he was awakened. This was one of the first and most graphic examples of correspondence between eye movements and dream report.

Figure 9: Sleep Apnea

This is a sample taken from the allnight recording of a patient with *sleep apnea*. From the beginning to the end of the sample is six minutes. The tracing marked RESP is hooked up in such a way that the pen moves down when the chest expands. In this remarkable example, there are only four episodes of breathing in the entire six minutes. Each episode consists of only three inspirations! No breathing occurs between episodes. These respiratory pauses are very long, lasting sixty to ninety seconds in contrast to the breathing episodes which last only five to ten seconds. This sample is from a REM period and the eye movements can be seen in the EOG tracing. Just prior to each group of three breaths, the patient *wakes up*. This can be seen as increased activity in the EMG (muscle activity) tracing. The most dramatic measurement in this example is from a device (O₂ SAT—top tracing) that registers the amount of oxygen in the blood. Note the large swings in the tracing. The peaks represent nearly normal oxygenation which is momentarily achieved when the patient wakes up and breathes. But, since he goes right back to sleep and stops breathing, the oxygen level immediately begins to fall. The scale is logarhythmic so that tiny differences toward the bottom are the same as big deviations toward the top. What this means is that oxygen in the blood keeps falling (it does not level off as the logarhythmic tracing appears to suggest) until it reaches a very low level which fortunately causes the patient to wake up and resume breathing. Try to imagine what it must be like to never sleep more than a minute or two at a time. Actually, this patient thought his sleep was normal. He had reached the point of becoming so used to the arousals and going back to sleep so quickly that he didn't remember any of them. However, he was overwhelmingly sleepy during the daytime, which was a consequence of the unsuspected nocturnal sleep disturbance. Some patients never get completely used to the arousals and, although they do not know they stop breathing, they do know their sleep is disturbed. These patients will complain of insomnia. The patient whose recording we have illustrated complained of hypersomnia.

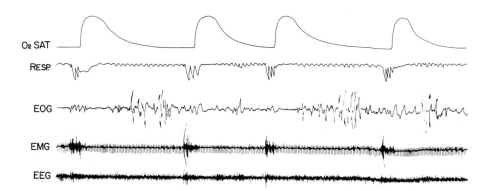

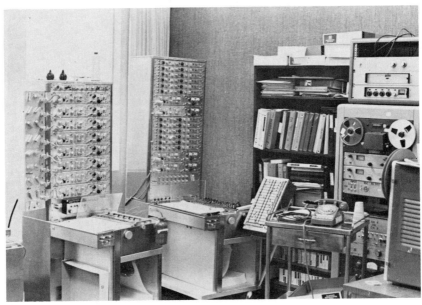

A

B

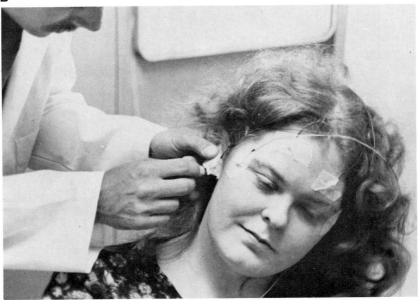

Figure 10:   Scenes from a Typical Sleep Laboratory

A. A large number of electronic instruments are needed for the study of physiological variables during sleep. The basic unit is the ink-writing oscillograph, which yields the miles of paper used in standard all-night or 24-hour sleep recordings. Tape recorders are needed to store data. Other special equipment stimulates the sleepers, draws blood continuously, analyzes breath-to-breath amounts of carbon dioxide, and makes others kinds of measurements.

B. A volunteer subject or a patient sits on a stool while the sleep-recording technician (called a "Polysomnographic Specialist" at the Stanford Sleep Disorders Clinic) attaches the small electrodes that will pick up the bioelectric signals during the test. Every attempt is made to minimize discomfort or distraction caused by these attachments. All the recording equipment is located outside the bedroom.

C. A subject is in bed, alseep. His posture is not important. Some subjects bury their faces in or under their pillows. The small bundle of lead wires going to the lead box attached to the head of the bed is long enough that the subject can move in a completely unrestricted manner or even sit up. An important goal is to make the subject feel completely at ease and to eliminate any sense of feeling "trapped." Subjects and patients are told that they are even free to disconnect themselves, by pulling the wires out of the lead box, if they feel an urgent desire to end a session in the laboratory.

C

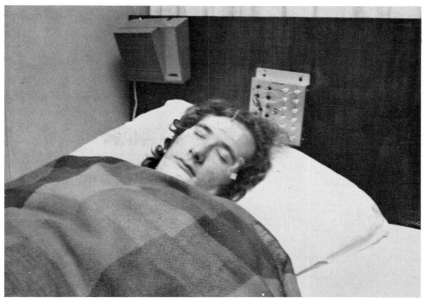

GLOSSARY

Alpha rhythm. A typical brain-wave pattern seen in relaxed wakefulness, characterized by continuous or waxing and waning sinusoidal fluctuations at or about ten cycles per second.

Autonomic nervous system. The part of the vertebrate nervous system that innervates smooth and cardiac muscle and glandular tissues and governs involuntary actions.

Axon. The elongated fiber that extends from the nerve cell but is part of it and conducts the nerve impulse; the axon usually branches many times before it terminates. (*See* Neuron.)

BRAC (basic rest-activity cycle). A term first used by Nathaniel Kleitman to describe a period of alternative quietude and activity in infants with a mean time of about sixty minutes. Kleitman found the activity portion of the cycle was either alert wakefulness or an interval of sleep in which numerous body movements were evident. Infants on self-demand feeding schedules seemed to want food at times that are integral multiples of the BRAC. We now know that during lengthy periods of continuous sleep, the part of the BRAC in which there is body movement corresponds to REM sleep. It is therefore clear that in newborn infants a considerable amount of body movement initiated in the brain breaks through the inhibitions imposed by REM sleep. Kleitman feels that the sixty-minute BRAC in infants generally lengthens to become the ninety-minute NREM-REM sleep cycle in the adult. Whether or not the ninety-minute BRAC really continues in some covert form during the day when humans are continuously awake is not known at the present time.

Brain stem. The part of the neuraxis, located at the base of the brain, that connects the spinal cord with the rest of the brain; it is thought to contain the mechanisms that regulate sleep-waking behavior. Many neuroanatomists say the brain stem consists of the mesencephalon, the pons, and the medulla oblongata.

Cataplexy. A sudden attack of complete or partial muscular paralysis precipitated by a strong emotion.

Central nervous system. The part of the nervous system that is housed within the bony cavities of the cranium and spinal column.

Circadian rhythm. Descriptive of cyclic biologic periods or rhythms having a time of about 24 hours. (*See Figure 2.*)

Cornea. The anterior part of the eyeball; specifically, the transparent covering of the iris.

Crib death syndrome. Describes cases in which infants in their first year of life are put to bed and are later found dead, presumably having died in their sleep. No cause of death can be found at autopsy.

Delirium tremens. A mental state characterized by illusions, hallucinations, short unsystematized delusions, excitement, restlessness, and incoherence, having a comparatively short course and accompanied often with tremors and shakiness. This state frequently follows acute alcoholic withdrawal.

Delta waves. High-amplitude, slow fluctuations in the brain-wave patterns; the amplitudes are greater than 75 microvolts and the frequencies are fewer than four cycles per second. (*See* Stage 4.)

Diencephalon. The part of the brain above the mesencephalon containing the thalamus, hypothalamus, and the geniculate bodies. (*See* Geniculate bodies; Mesencephalon.)

EEG (electroencephalogram). The recording of brain activity made by an electroencephalograph.

EMG (electromyogram). The polygraph record of muscle activity showing electrical potentials generated in the muscle fibers.

Enuresis. Bed-wetting. This sleep disorder occurs almost exclusively in young children.

EOG (electrooculogram). The polygraph record of eye movement.

ESP (extrasensory perception). Transmission of information from one person to another by means other than the ordinary physical sensory channels. Also known as telepathy.

Geniculate bodies, Lateral. A dense cluster of cell bodies in the thalamus (diencephalon) that send axons to the visual cortex and receive axons directly from ganglion cells of the retina of the eye. Thus, the lateral geniculate bodies are the first way station in the visual system. In this area in the brain of the cat high-amplitude waves, or spikes, have been recorded. (*See* PGO spikes.)

Hallucinations, Hypnagogic. Vivid, often frightening dreams that occur at the onset of sleep.

Hypersomnia. The complaint of too much sleep, or of feeling sleepy all the time despite a normal or excessive amount of sleep at night. The complaint is not always confirmed by sleep laboratory studies. In a general sense, it means excessive sleep.

Hypnotic compounds. Sleeping pills.

Insomnia. Complaint of too little sleep.

Insomnia, Idiopathic. Insomnia without known cause.

Insomnia, Pseudo-. The complaint of disturbed sleep despite essentially normal sleep patterns in all-night sleep-recordings.

Intercostal Muscles. Muscles between the ribs arranged in such a way that their contraction serves to raise or lower the rib cage.

Jet-lag syndrome. Describes a brief maladjustment experienced when an abrupt change in the length of a day causes "body time" or circadian rhythm to be out of phase temporarily with "clock time."

K complexes. A term that designates a paroxysmal wave-form of high amplitude standing out from a low-amplitude background in the EEG. K complexes may occur either spontaneously or in response to a stimulus. (*See Figure 4.*)

LOC (left outer canthus). *See* ROC.

Medulla oblongata. The truncated cone of nervous tissue that is continuous to the pons above it and to the spinal cord below it. It lies ventral to the cerebellum and its upper surface forms the floor of the fourth ventricle.

Mesencephalon (midbrain). Part of the brain stem above the pons and below the diencephalon. The mesencephalon is thought by some to form the upper part and limit of the brain stem.

Microsleep. A lapse or block in normal waking behavior often associated with a change of brain waves from waking patterns to sleep patterns. Microsleep usually lasts only a few seconds, during which an external stimulus will not be detected by the subject.

Monoamine oxidase inhibitors. Drugs that inhibit the enzyme monoamine oxidase, which is the main agent that breaks down the biogenic amine compounds serotonin and noradrenalin; such inhibition leads to an increase in the amounts of these compounds in the brain.

Myoclonias. Conditions characterized by shock-like contractions of a part of an entire muscle or a group of muscles. The sudden starts at the onset of sleep are usually accompanied by a single myoclonic jerk, or by several. The muscle twitches during REM sleep are sometimes included in this category.

Narcolepsy. An illness typified by "sleep attacks" and/or excessive sleepiness during the day, together with peculiar attacks of muscular weakness and/or paralysis precipitated by strong emotion (cataplexy). Narcolepsy can be identified, in laboratory studies, by evidence of passage from wakefulness directly into REM sleep. Thus, the "sleep attack" of narcolepsy is an attack of REM sleep. The term is used imprecisely by many to refer to any condition of excessive sleepiness.

Neonatal sleep. Pertaining to the sleep of infants in the first four weeks after birth.

Neuron. A specialized cell that forms the basic unit of the nervous system. The neuron usually has a cell body, complex receptive appendages called dendrites, and a single elongated filament (the axon) that usually branches many times before termination at the synapse, where it connects with other receptive elements.

NREM sleep (pronounced non-REM). Essentially all the sleep remaining after REM sleep is subtracted; a sleep in which there are no rapid eye movements. Brain-wave patterns during NREM sleep generally show slow waves and spindles; muscle tone is preserved. (*See* Stage 1; Stage 2; Stage 3; Stage 4; *Figure 4.*)

Nucleus locus coeruleus. A cluster of noradrenalin-containing cells in the pons thought to contain mechanisms relating to REM sleep. (*See Figure 1.*)

Nucleus subcoeruleus. A cluster of cells just under the nucleus locus coeruleus.

Occipital cortex. The part of the neocortex of the brain, posterior and basal, that receives and processes visual information. PGO spikes are recorded in this area in the cat during REM sleep.

Pavor nocturnis. "Night terrors," which occur almost exclusively in children. Episodes of this sleep disorder arise from the depths of the first Stage 4 sleep of night and are generally associated with intense body movements and intense autonomic activity.

PCPA (parachlorophenylalanine). A compound, similar in structure to the amino acid phenylalanine, that inhibits or blocks the conversion of the amino acid tryptophan to 5-hydroxytryptophan. Since 5-hydroxytryptophan is the immediate precursor of serotonin, serotonin is not formed in the brain in the presence of PCPA and the amount of serotonin present in the brain decreases as it is used up by nerve activity. (*See* Serotonin.)

PGO spike. A dramatic wave-form recorded during REM sleep and produced, in the brain of the cat, by the electrical activity in specific places; namely the pons, the geniculate bodies, and the occipital cortex. The initial wave-form is a monophasic spike of high amplitude lasting about 50 milliseconds. A few PGO spikes are also seen in the NREM sleep of cats. The interest in the spikes derives from the fact that they are closely related to rapid eye movements and muscle twitches in the cat. Some people think PGO spikes might constitute the neurological basis of dreaming, because the wave-form seems to be generated in the pons and thence to ascend the visual pathways. However, PGO spikes have not been directly observed in man. (*See* Geniculate bodies; Occipital cortex; Pons.)

PIP (phasic integrated potential). A recording of the electrical potential of muscle fibers near the eye, electronically amplified and integrated. Since activity is very brief, the recording resembles a spike thought to be a human analogue of PGO waves in the cat. (*See* PGO spikes.)

Polygraph. An instrument for simultaneously recording tracings of several different physiological variables.

Pons. The smallest part of the brain stem, lying between the medulla oblongata and the mesencephalon. The pons is perhaps the most crucial part of the brain stem with regard to sleep and wakefulness. It contains raphe neurons and locus coeruleus neurons.

Raphe nuclei. A complex of nine narrow cellular clusters on the exact midline that extends through the length of the brain stem (*see Figure 1*). The cells in these clusters are thought to contain serotonin. (*See* Serotonin.)

REM rebound. The characteristic increase in the time of REM sleep following a prior reduction.

REM sleep. A unique state of sleep found in nearly all mammals, including man, during which the activity of the brain approximates the activity observed in the alert waking state, and during which there is an active motor inhibition or paralysis of voluntary muscles. In cats, the brain-wave patterns of REM sleep resemble exactly those observed in wakefulness; in man, saw-tooth brain-wave patterns are observed. The motor paralysis is revealed in the suppression recorded in EMGs. (*See* Saw-tooth waves.)

Reticular formation. The central neuronal network (reticulum) of the brain stem, in which are housed many of the sleep and wakefulness mechanisms. Nuclei (dense clusters of neurons) are often not clearly defined.

Retina. The back part of the eyeball, which contains the light receptors and is continuous to the optic nerve.

ROC (right outer canthus). The corner of the eye is called the canthus. The abbreviation generally identifies an electrode placed on the facial skin as near the right outer canthus as possible. LOC refers to the left outer canthus, and to the electrode placed there.

Saw-tooth waves. Wave-forms seen uniquely in the EEGs of humans during REM periods (*see bottom tracing in Figure 4.*) They tend to occur in bursts of two to three cycles at a rate of two to three per second and often precede or overlap a burst of rapid eye movements.

Scanning hypothesis. The notion that the temporal-spatial pattern of rapid eye movements in REM sleep is related to the specific unfolding visual imagery of a dream, as if the eyes were moving to scan the hallucinatory images of a dream.

Schizophrenics. Persons afflicted with a psychotic condition characterized by a splitting of the mental functions. Such people often experience hallucinations.

Serotonin. The compound found in the cell bodies and terminals of neurons located in the Raphe complex that is thought to be a neurotransmitter; the compound that, when released, transmits and stimulates the post-synaptic neuron. Serotonin is a biogenic amine with an indole nucleus made from the dietary amino acid tryptophan in two steps—hydroxylation and decarboxylation.

Sleep apnea. A respiratory failure seemingly induced by sleep or associated only with sleep.

Sleep cycle, Basic ninety-minute. Characteristically, NREM and REM sleep alternate through the night. The first sleep cycle is one lasting from sleep onset to the end of the first REM period; the second sleep cycle is measured from the end of the first REM period to the end of the second REM period; and so forth. When all cycles are totalled and averaged, their mean value is near ninety minutes for young adults.

Sleep spindle. A typical wave-form seen in EEGs during NREM sleep and characterized by a burst of very regular oscillations at a frequency of from 12 to 14 cycles per second. Sleep spindles are observed oftenest during NREM EEG Stage 2, but they may also be seen in Stage 4 when the slow waves are filtered out.

Stage 1. A kind of NREM sleep defined in the EEG by patterns not containing alpha waves, sleep spindles, or high-amplitude waves. Generally a transitional stage. *(See Figure 4.)*

Stage 2. A kind of NREM sleep defined in the EEG by the presence of sleep spindles and K complexes. The background patterns are low in their amplitude *(see Figure 4)*. The largest part of NREM sleep in young adults is Stage 2.

Stage 3. A kind of NREM sleep defined in the EEG by the presence of a small amount of high-amplitude, slow waves. Generally Stage 3 is a transition between Stage 2 and Stage 4. *(See Figure 4.)*

Stage 4. A kind of NREM sleep defined in the EEG by a predominance of high-amplitude, slow waves (delta waves). *(See Figure 4.)*

Wakefulness. The state of being awake, measurable with characteristic brain-wave patterns that are dominated either by alpha rhythm or low-amplitude high-frequency (greater than ten cycles per second) rhythms.

READER'S GUIDE

Inside Information

Although most people have some awareness of the vast proliferation of scientific literature currently published worldwide (there are some 80,000 scientific journals), they probably think, if they consider it at all, that sleep comprises a narrow area of inquiry pursued by a few insomniac crackpots. On the contrary, sleep research is right in the proliferative mainstream—a respectable scientific calling (as I hope this book has portrayed). There is a vast amount of scientific literature which the investigator must follow, with a diffusion of both the literature and the practitioners. Not only must papers be read; they must first be located!

To better illustrate the extent of the problem, I would like to quote from a document that I wrote in 1969: "Sleep research shares with many other areas the problem posed by the avalanching volume of scientific publications. The sleep literature is tremendously disseminated. Statistics from the *Sleep Bulletin Annual Cumulation-1968* indicate that there were only eighteen journals in the world in which five or more articles on sleep appeared, whereas there were 158 journals in which four or fewer articles appeared. This dissemination makes it virtually impossible for the individual investigator to follow the sleep and dreaming literature closely. This difficulty is compounded by the number of languages involved."

Furthermore, at present there is no single journal solely devoted to sleep literature. To cope with problems in this and other areas, the National Institute of Neurological Diseases and Stroke has established a neurological information network in which many major academic centers participate. One of the most important services is the UCLA

Brain Information Service, which was established in the Brain Research Institute and Biomedical Library of UCLA. As part of its several services, it publishes monthly the *Sleep Bulletin*, mentioned above, a compilation of all scientific articles in the area of sleep and dreams with the exception of purely psychological articles. The BIS also publishes *Sleep Reviews*, a monthly selection of critical reviews of sleep literature. I was founding editor of *Sleep Reviews*, although I have since passed the reins to David Foulkes. Annually the monthly issues of *Sleep Bulletin* are compiled and put out as a year's selection. *Anyone* is eligible to receive *Sleep Bulletin* and *Sleep Reviews*, and need only request them from the Brain Information Service, University of California at Los Angeles, Los Angeles, California 90024. Annual compilations dating back to 1969 are available. Michael Chase, the inestimable director of the Brain Information Service, now publishes annual volumes entitled *Sleep Research* that contain the annual compilations as well as abstracts of APPS meetings. There is also a bibliography available from the Brain Information Service, compiled by Allan Rechtschaffen and Doty Eakin, which includes literature from 1964 through 1967.

Scientific Meetings

Another kind of insider's note is the fact that many of you who have wanted to attend scientific meetings of particular interest to you may do so in the field of sleep research. The difficulties of being admitted to scientific meetings vary from group to group. For example, in recent years gaining admittance to the national convention of the American Medical Association has required passing a security check that rivals that of the national Democratic or Republican conventions. On the other hand, some groups are entirely open, but apparently of little general interest, with audiences of ten or twelve persons seated in the vast emptiness of a hotel auditorium. The society which fosters scientific communication in the sleep and dream area is known as the Association for the Psychophysiological Study of Sleep, or APSS. Allan Rechtschaffen and I founded this group in 1961 and the first meeting was held at the University of Chicago. We have never restricted attendance; we have never imposed any barrier, other than the limit of time itself, on anyone who has anything of substance to say and wishes to present a paper; we have never checked credentials. In short, while we do not publicly invite the press and public, we readily welcome those who chose to attend. The 1973 meeting of the APSS was held in May in San Diego. A Stanford alumnus, Dr. Laverne Johnson, was the program chairman of this session.

Best Buy

One of the chief problems in suggesting reading material from such a very young and very active field is that the material quickly becomes obsolete. As new light is shed on the vast areas of ignorance, today's exciting hypothesis becomes tomorrow's foolishness. Moreover, in spite of the intrinsic interest of the subject, there are very few popular books about sleep, and virtually none by professional researchers.

Undoubtedly, one of the most up-to-date general coverages of the subject is a book soon to be marketed by the Brain Information Service. Michael Chase has edited a volume which is the result of a series of symposia held at the first International Congress of the APSS in June 1971, in Bruges, Belgium. The book, *The Sleeping Brain*, has among its contributors the foremost authorities on sleep and dream research. In contrast to usual symposia in which a series of highly egocentric chapters are published referring to an individual's work, each chapter in *The Sleeping Brain* is the author's summary of ten or twelve experts' thoughts on a specific area. It includes sections on "Foundations of the Sleep States," "Patterns within the Sleep States," and "Alterations of the Sleep States." At the cost of $15 ($13, soft cover; Calif. residents add 6% sales tax), the book will be available soon from the Brain Research Institute Publications Office, UCLA Center for Health Sciences, Los Angeles, California 90024. A poster of the delightful cover of the book may be obtained from the same source at $1 per copy (Calif. residents add 6% sales tax). If the reader is going to read any scientific book at all, there is some advantage in reading the most up-to-date, and I highly recommend *The Sleeping Brain*.

Readings

There is a vast gulf between the sensational articles (Dream and Stay Sane) of the newsstand periodicals and the scientific literature on sleep and dreams. There are almost no sensible popular books on sleep, books which it would not be a disservice to recommend. Very few of the scholarly treatments can justifiably be called popular. I will make specific recommendations with comments, and then list a number of "also recommended" books and articles.

General—Sleep and Dreaming

In my opinion, one I am sure is shared by many others, the work which is at once the most scholarly and best written in the field of sleep and dreams is the monograph by Nathaniel Kleitman entitled *Sleep and Wakefulness* (revised and enlarged edition, Chicago: University of Chicago Press, 1963). I cut my teeth on the first edition of this book, published in 1939, and I recall it as effortless to read—an unusual property of a monograph of this size. I am sure the reader could easily feel a sense of pride in reading a volume that is so complete in its presentation of the topic. Nathaniel Kleitman now is retired and living in Santa Monica and is a regular consultant to our laboratory, visiting at least twice a year. I quote from the foreword to the first edition, which suggests a style not common among modern technologically oriented scientists: "Since my own reading ability is limited to French, German, Italian, and Russian, I was fortunate in securing the assistance of B. B. Lifshultz, whose knowledge of the Scandinavian languages as well as Dutch and Spanish was an invaluable help to me in gathering and classifying the bibliographic material." The revised edition, which is a product of unremitting effort on the part of Professor Kleitman, contains the important sleep literature from 1912 through May 1962. It also includes references to 100 pre-1912 classical papers which were previously omitted.

One of the first popular books from the post-REM era, and in my opinion one of the best, was written by Edwin Diamond and called *The Science of Dreams* (New York: Doubleday, 1962). Ed Diamond was then the scientific editor of *Newsweek* and was responsible for the magazine's cover story on sleep and dream research. His book covers a wide area and includes sociological and anthropological work, Freudian theories, and laboratory studies. It is well written and, although somewhat dated, well worth reading.

Another especially recommended book, of which I was unaware until it came to me as a Christmas gift last year from an unusually discerning young lady, is called *Journey Into Night, An Anthology of the Night in Words and Pictures*, which was compiled by H. J. Deverson (London: Leslie Frewin, 1966). It is particularly good in evoking the literary and in considering the vast differences between day and night and what they mean to all aspects of human activity. Sample chapter headings are "Night is for Pleasure," "Night is for Dreams," "Night is for Sleep," "Night is for the Sleepless," "Night is for Witches," "Night is for Beds," "Night is for Owls," and "Night is for Love."

The most detailed and authentic popular book on sleep that one still sees on the shelves of bookstores is *Sleep*, by Gay Luce and Julius Segal (New York: Lancer, 1966). One of the few popularizations by a professional is *Sleep*, by Ian Oswald (Middlesex, England: Penguin Books, 1966). Oswald has also written a more scholarly work entitled *Sleeping and Waking* (New York: Elsevier, 1962).

There are several popular articles that give a flavor of the sleep laboratory. The first of these is a profile that appeared in the *New*

Yorker, by Calvin Trilling. This excellent writer spent several days in our laboratory in early 1965 and wrote a lengthy "reporter at large" article entitled "A Third State of Existence" which was published September 18, 1965. The other two articles were written by me and published at Stanford: "Through the Door of Dreams" in *Stanford Today*, Series 1, Vol. 12, 1965; and "A New Look at the Third State of Existence," *Stanford M.D.*, Vol. 8, No. 1, 1968-69.

I think that a very good introduction to the subject of sleep and dreaming is my own lengthy article, "An Essay on Dreams," which accounts for about one-fourth of the book *New Directions in Psychology II* (New York: Holt, Rinehart and Winston, 1965), which is available in most college bookstores.

I would also strongly recommend the following which are slightly more scholarly but very readable, general books on sleep and dreaming:

Abt, L.E., and B.F. Riess (eds.). *Dreams and Dreaming*. Progress in Clinical Psychology. Vol. VIII. New York: Grune and Stratton, 1968.

Hartmann, E. (ed.). *Sleep and Dreaming*. International Psychiatry Clinic. Vol. VII. Boston: Little, Brown, 1970.

Kales, A. (ed.). *Sleep—Physiology and Pathology: A Symposium*. Philadelphia: J.B. Lippincott, 1969.

Webb, W.B. *Sleep: An Experimental Approach*. New York: Macmillan, 1968.

Witkin, H.A., and H.B. Lewis (eds.). *Experimental Studies of Dreaming*. New York: Random House, 1967.

Physiological and Biochemical

These references are for the reader who is interested in the more scientific aspects of sleep. Perhaps the most up-to-date and authoritative is a review by my friend, Michel Jouvet, "The Role of Monoamines and Acetylcholine-Containing Neurons in the Regulation of the Sleep-Waking Cycle" (in *Reviews of Physiology, Biochemistry and Experimental Pharmacology*. New York: Springer-Verlag, 1972). This is easily the most readable in English of the articles by the French scientist.

Another review that is worthwhile is by Werner P. Koella, entitled *Sleep—Its Nature and Physiological Organization* (Springfield, Ill.: C.C. Thomas, 1967).

Also recommended are:

Clemente, C.D. (ed.). "The Physiological Correlates of Dreaming," *Experimental Neurology*. Supplement 4. New York: Academic Press, 1967.

Hartmann, E. *The Biology of Dreaming.* Springfield, Ill.: C.C. Thomas, 1967.

Magoun, H.W. *The Waking Brain,* 2d ed. Springfield, Ill.: C.C. Thomas, 1963.

Wolstenholme, G.E.W., and M. O'Connor (eds.). *CIBA Foundation Symposium on the Nature of Sleep.* Boston: Little, Brown, 1960.

Dreams and Dreaming

Although quite a bit of information on dreaming is sprinkled throughout the books listed above, perhaps the best book which deals with dreaming and takes the laboratory findings into account is *The Psychology of Sleep* by David Foulkes (New York: Charles Scribner's Sons, 1966). Another book, edited by Milton Kramer, is entitled *Dream Psychology and the New Biology of Dreaming* (Springfield, Ill.: C.C. Thomas, 1969).

Content analysis is probably the most objective way of approaching the study of dream content. From this point of view, two books by Calvin Hall are recommended. An early one which was derived from Hall's accumulation of about 10,000 dreams is called *The Meaning of Dreams* (New York: Dell, 1959). A second, more technical book which he co-authored with Robert Van de Castle is *The Content Analysis of Dreams* (New York: Appleton-Century-Crofts, 1966).

The granddaddy of them all with regard to the meaning of dreams is, of course, Sigmund Freud's *The Interpretation of Dreams* (London: Allen & Unwin, 1954; first printing, 1900). By virtue of both his exceptionally clear exposition and excellent translation, this book is marvelously readable. It is the foundation of what is still the most important approach to the meaning (if any) of dreams. A companion volume to this, and one which is quite interesting, is *The New Psychology of Dreaming* by Richard M. Jones (New York: Grune and Stratton, 1970), which deals with modern psychoanalytic theory of dreaming in light of laboratory findings.

Jung's theories are dealt with in two volumes which are available in paperback editions:

Jung, C.G. *Modern Man in Search of a Soul.* London: Paul, Trench, Trubner, 1933.

————. *Memories, Dreams, Reflections,* A. Faffe (ed.). New York: Random House, 1961.

There are two older books which are quite good. The first is by Havelock Ellis, who is familiar to many students of psychology as an early writer on human sexuality. Ellis wrote a delightful book called *The World of Dreams* (Boston: Houghton Mifflin, 1911). The other book is a marvelous anthology edited by Ralph L. Woods, also entitled *The World of Dreams* (New York: Random House, 1947).

One of the most beautiful books on dreams and dreaming, covering a wide range of topics, is *Dreams and Dreaming* by N. Mackenzie (London: Aldus Books, 1965). This book is full of remarkable illustrations, some in color. A *must* for anyone who collects this literature.

Also recommended are the following books which are either specialized or idiosyncratic in their viewpoint:

Arnold-Forster, H.O. *Studies in Dreams.* New York: Macmillan, 1921. (An account of the author's adventures after she learned to "control" her dreams.)

Breger, L., I. Hunter, and R. W. Lane. *The Effect of Stress on Dreams.* New York: International Universities Press, 1971.

Hadfield, J.A. *Dreams and Nightmares.* London: Penguin Books, 1954.

Jones, E. *On the Nightmare.* London: Hogarth Press, 1949.

Kettelkamp, L. *Dreams.* New York: William Morrow, 1968. (This is a book for your little children.)

Kimmins, C.W. *Children's Dreams—An Unexplored Land.* New York: W.W. Norton, 1937.

Lowes, J.L. *The Road to Xanadu.* New York: Vintage Books, 1959. (This book, in recalling the story of Kubla Khan coming to Coleridge in a dream, deals with .the creative unconscious process.)

Malcolm, N. *Dreaming*, R.F. Holland (ed.). New York: Humanities Press, 1959.

Roheim, G. *The Eternal Ones of the Dream.* New York: International Universities Press, 1969.

———. *The Gates of the Dream.* New York: International Universities Press, 1952.

Singer, J.L. *Daydreaming.* New York: Random House, 1966.

Sonnet, A. *The Twilight Zone of Dreams.* Rahway, New Jersey: Quinn & Boden, 1961. (This book deals with creativity and dreams and tells many apocryphal stories. It should be read almost as fiction.)

Van Grunebaum, G.E., and R. Caillois (eds.). *The Dream and Human Societies.* Berkeley: University of California Press, 1966.

Finally, one should read at least one book of the many which are available on bookstands that are, in effect, code books translating dream symbols into their appropriate meanings. For example, in *The Dream Dictionary* by I. Woolever, there are such things as: if you dream of oil, you have been the victim of a slippery operator; if you dream of an oyster, it means sexual fulfillment; if you dream of peaches, it means health and good fortune; and so on. These are, of course, patent nonsense, but somehow rather interesting. The earliest of such volumes of dream interpretation was the *Oneirocritica*, by Artemidorus, written in the second century.

I cannot recommend any book which deals specifically with things like sleep deprivation, but an excellent article by Williams, Lubin, and Goodnow, "Impaired Performance in Acute Sleep Loss" (*Psychological Monographs, 73*: 1-26, 1959), is one of the landmarks in the field.

Also recommended are:

> Wilkinson, R.T. "Sleep Deprivation," *Physiology of Human Survival*, O.G. Edholme (ed.). New York: Academic Press, 1965.

> Van de Castle, R. *The Psychology of Dreaming*. New York: General Learning Press, 1971.

Pharmacology of Sleep

In this category I would recommend two very scholarly reviews:

> King, C.D. "The pharmacology of rapid eye movement sleep," *Advances in Pharmacology and Chemotherapy, 9*: 1-91, 1971.

> Oswald, I. "Drugs and Sleep," *Pharmacological Review, 20*: 273-303, 1968.

Sleep Disorders

At the present time the best book in this area that one could recommend for the general reader is *Insomnia: The Guide for Troubled Sleepers*, by Luce and Segal (Garden City, N.Y.: Doubleday, 1969). Most of the other popular books are probably likely to do more harm than good.

Information about new insights into the role of sleeping pills has not been widely disseminated, but articles by Anthony Kales are recommended as well as those by Oswald.

The best scholarly work in this area is *The Abnormalities of Sleep in Man* edited by H. Gastuat, E. Lugaresi, G. Berti Ceroni, and G. Coccagna (Proceedings of the XVth European Meeting on Electroencephalography. Bologna: Aulo Gaggi, 1968). A new book will soon be coming out on periodic respiration (sleep apnea) by Lugaresi.

Finally, I recommend a paper by Roger Broughton, "Sleep Disorders: Disorders of Arousal?" (*Science, 159*: 1070-78, 1968), which deals with things like sleepwalking, sleep talking, and so on.

Circadian Rhythms

Especially recommended for popular reading is a new book by Gay Gaer Luce entitled *Body Time* (New York: Random House, 1971).

Another popular book written by M. Siffre, who spent several months in a cave, is *Beyond Time* (New York: McGraw–Hill, 1964). A recent article in the *New Yorker* by M. Tiden tells about experiences in Tromsö, Norway ("A Reporter at Large," March 18, 1972).

Also recommended are:

Aschoff, J. (ed.). *Circadian Clocks*. Amsterdam: North Holland Publishing, 1965.

Conroy, R., and J.M. Mills. *Human Circadian Rhythms*. Baltimore: Williams and Wilkins, 1971.

Kleitman, N., and H. Kleitman. "The sleep-wakefulness pattern in the Arctic," *Scientific Monthly,* 76: 349-56, 1953.

Mills, J.N. (ed.). *Biological Aspects of Circadian Rhythms*. London: Plenum Press, 1971.

Richter, C.P. *Biological Clocks in Medicine and Psychiatry*. Springfield, Ill.: C.C. Thomas, 1965.

Sollberger, A. *Biological Rhythm Research*. Amsterdam/London/New York: Elsevier Publishing, 1965.

Ward, R.R. *The Living Clocks*. New York: Knopf, 1971.

Sleep and Dreams in Mental Illness

This is an area in which I have been very interested and I would recommend several papers from my own pen:

Dement, W., C. Halper, *et al.* "Hallucinations and Dreaming," *Res. Publ. Assoc. Res. Nerv. Ment. Dis., 48:* 335-59, 1970.

———, V. Zarcone, *et al.* "Some parallel findings in schizophrenic patients and serotonin-depleted cats," *Schizophrenia—Current Concepts and Research*, D.V. Siva Sankar (ed.). Hicksville, N.Y.: PJD Publications, 1969.

Sleep Deprivation Illness

This is a very active area and there are many interesting findings; however, most of them are very technical. There are two basic concepts. One is the notion that sleep deprivation leads to mental illness, which does not appear to be strictly true. On this point of view:

Gulevich, G., W. Dement, and I. Johnson. "Psychiatric and EEG observations on a case of prolonged (264 hours) wakefulness," *Archives of General Psychiatry, 15:* 29-35, 1966.

Kales, A., *et al.* "Sleep patterns following 205 hours of sleep deprivation," *Psychosomatic Medicine, 32:* 189-200, 1970.

The second concept is the notion that a dream is a psychosis. At this point, since everyone has had direct experience of dreaming, the most helpful thing is an understanding of psychosis and schizophrenia. I think there are three marvelous books in this area. One, by Hannah Green, *I Never Promised You a Rose Garden* (New York: New American Library, Inc., 1964), was a best seller. An incredibly well-written and fascinating book, one of the most outstanding in the history of psychiatry, is *Dementia Praecox or the Group of Schizophrenias* by Eugen Bleuler (New York: International Universities Press, 1952). Finally, there is an excellent compilation by Carney Landis, edited by Fred Mettler, called *The Varieties of Psychopathological Experience* (New York: Holt, Rinehart & Winston, 1964).

Miscellaneous

Among the older books which I recommend as interesting reading is M. de Manaceine, *Sleep: Its Physiology, Pathology, Hygiene and Psychology* (New York: Charles Scribner's Sons, 1909). For those who can read French, I would suggest H. Pieron's *Le Probleme Physiologique du Sommeil* (Paris: Masson & Cie, 1913), which has some information on the evolution of sleep which is generally unavailable.

It is quite likely that transcendental meditation is related to the physiology we see just at the onset of sleep. A young psychologist, Robert K. Wallace, has had his thesis on this subject published as *The Physiological Effects of Transcendental Meditation* (Los Angeles: Student's International Meditation Society, 1970).

Also recommended are:

Bertini, M. (ed.). *Psicofisiologia del Sonno e del Sogno*. Proceedings of an International Symposium, Rome, 1967. Milan: Editrice Vita e Pensiero, 1970.

Hamburg, D.A., K.H. Pribram, and A.J. Steinkard (eds.). *Perception and its Disorders*. Baltimore: Williams and Wilkins, 1970.

Hilgard, E.R., with a chapter by J.R. Hilgard. *Hypnotic Susceptibility*. New York: Harcourt-Brace-World, 1965.

Jouvet, M. (ed.). *Neurophysiologie des Etats du Sommeil*. Paris: Centre National de la Recherche Scientifique, 1965.

Madow, L., and L.H. Snow (eds.). *The Psychodynamic Implications of the Physiological Studies on Dreams*. Springfield, Ill.: C.C. Thomas, 1970.

Tart, C.T. (ed.) *Altered States of Consciousness: A Book of Readings*. New York: Wiley, 1969.

Movies

There are a number of interesting films about sleep which range from depicting the techniques of sleep research to illustrating sleep disorders. They may either be purchased outright, or rented or borrowed, depending upon their original distribution. The following movies are available to the public:

To Sleep . . . Perchance to Dream, produced by Harold Mayer, directed by Al Swerdloff. This film was one of the first to be made in the modern era of sleep research and was shown on National Educational Television in 1966. The project was funded by the National Institute of Mental Health and the film is available from Harold Mayer Productions, Inc., in New York City. The film includes sleep experiments by Drs. Kleitman, Kales, and me at UCLA.

The Sleeping Brain, produced by Dr. James B. Maas and Anne D. Cook in collaboration with Dr. Michel Jouvet, 1971. This film explores the neurophysiology and neuropsychology of sleep and dreaming. Research methodology is demonstrated through a series of experiments on cats. Although you may find it a little gory in parts, this is an excellent film. It is available from Houghton Mifflin Co., Boston, Mass.

Sleeping and Dreaming in Humans, produced by Dr. James B. Maas and Anne D. Cook in collaboration with Dr. William C. Dement, 1971. In this movie, I demonstrate the techniques and methodology of human sleep research. It is also available from Houghton Mifflin.

Narcolepsy, produced in the Stanford University Sleep Disorders Clinic, 1971. This film depicts the symptoms of narcolepsy and includes some discussion by me and Dr. Vincent P. Zarcone with some of our narcoleptic patients. This film was funded by Hoffman-LaRoche, Nutley, New Jersey, and is available through that organization.

Exploring Serotonin, produced by Mr. Edmund Levy of the Health Learning Systems, 1972. This film covers the recent work in our laboratory and includes a discussion by Dr. Richard Wyatt of the National Institute of Mental Health. It is primarily about serotonin and sleep, PCPA, schizophrenia and 5HTP. The film is available from Pfizer Laboratories, New York City, which funded the project.

Sleep Disorders, produced by Squibb Laboratories, 1972. This film was only recently completed and it contains my discussion of sleep disorders. It will be available from Squibb Laboratories, Princeton, New Jersey.

A Decade Full of Dreams, produced by John Glick and Bill Gonda. In my opinion, this film is more entertaining than educational. The producers are both sons of Stanford Medical School faculty members and both worked in my lab for many years. *Decade* is a very in-group movie and was intended to make the 10th Annual Meeting of the APSS a memorable occasion. The film is a delightful, light-hearted farce that ostensibly chronicles ten years of sleep research. The musical sound track adds immeasurably to the enjoyment of the movie.

INDEX

measurement of, *Fig. 3*
and REM sleep, 26
Performance
  and circadian rhythm, 18
  and sleep deprivation, 8-9, 15
Perphenazine, 87
Personality disorders and sleep
    deprivation, 8
PGO spikes, 27, 51, 92
Phasic intergrated potential (PIP),
    27
Physical fitness and sleep deprivation,
    12
Pittendrigh, Colin, 18
Pivik, Terry, 51, 93
Placidyl (ethchlorvinol), 81
Polygraph, 22, 23, 24, 25, *Fig. 3*
Pons, 27, *Fig. 1*
Pregnancy and need for sleep, 4
Premature infants, REM sleep in, 30
Primitive cultures and dreams, 2-3
Prince, Morton, 97
Problem solving during sleep, 96,
    98-102
Prolonged wakefulness
  Guinness Record for, 9
  of Peter Tripp, 8, 87
  of Randy Gardner, 8-13, 87
  in rats, 12
Pseudoinsomnia, 82
Psychomotor performance and sleep
    deprivation, 8-9, 15
Psychosis
  schizophrenia, 55-56, 86-87, 92, 93
  and sleep deprivation, 8, 12

Raphe nuclei, *Fig. 1*
Rapid-eye-movement sleep. *See* REM
    sleep
Rats
  and prolonged wakefulness, 12
  REM sleep in, 30
Reaction speed and sleep deprivation,
    6
Rechtschaffen, Allan, 41, 71, 91
  on function of sleep, 16
  and narcolepsy, 77
  and NREM dream recall, 44, 65
  and PIP, 27
REM sleep, 24-33, 35-36, *Figs. 1, 3*

in animals, 30-31, 50
deprivation, 90-92
discovery of, 24-25
and dream content, 52-53, 66-68,
    71
and dream recall, 37-40, 44-45, 56,
    85, *Fig. 7*
and dream sequence, 59, 62-65
duration of, 36-37, *Fig. 5*
and narcoleptics, 77-78
in newborns, 26, 30-31, 51, 52-53,
    71
paralysis during, 26, 77-78
phasic activity in, 26-27
rebound, 80, 91, 92, 93
refractory period of, 36-37
saw-tooth waves, 28, 50, *Fig. 4*
and scanning hypothesis, 47-52
and serotonin, 92
and sleep apnea, *Fig. 9*
Reptiles, NREM sleep in, 30
Reserpine, 70
Respiration. *See* Breathing
Rest-activity cycle, basic. *See* BRAC
Rest versus sleep, 6
Reticular formation of brain stem, 14
Retina, 23
Rhodes, Jack, 50
Richardson, B. H., 21-22, *Fig. 6*
Ritalin, 78
RNA, messenger, 18
ROC (right outer canthus), *Fig. 8*
Roffwarg, Howard, 48-49, 51, 66, 70,
    Fig. 8
Royal, Royce, 15

San Diego Naval Hospital, 12
Saw-tooth waves, 28, 50, *Fig. 4*
Scanning hypothesis, 47-52, *Fig. 8*
Schizophrenics
  dreams of, 55-56
  sleep in, 93
  and sleeplessness, 86-87, 92
Sensory activity and sleep
    deprivation, 6
Sensory stimulation and wakefulness,
    13, 15-16
Serapis (Egyptian god of dreams), 2
Serotonergic neurons in brain stem,
    14, *Fig. 1*

ABOUT THE AUTHOR

Dr. William C. Dement was a second-year medical student at The University of Chicago and an employee in Professor Nathaniel Kleitman's sleep research laboratory in 1952 when Kleitman and his assistants made the first observations and descriptions of rapid-eye-movement sleep; it was Dr. Dement who coined the term "REM," now commonly used to refer to that phenomenon. Dr. Dement subsequently earned his M.D. and a Ph.D. in physiology from The University of Chicago and has pursued a distinguished career investigating the physiology of sleep and dreams.

Dr. Dement is cofounder of the Association for the Psychophysiological Study of Sleep, founding editor-in-chief of *Sleep Reviews*, and author of more than 150 scientific papers on sleep and dreams. In 1963 he established the Sleep Laboratory at Stanford University and in 1970 he founded the Stanford University Sleep Disorders Clinic, where he now serves as director. The clinic is devoted to diagnosis and treatment of disorders that disturb the sleep of millions of people. For his work in sleep research, Dr. Dement has been honored with the Thomas W. Salmon Medal of the New York Academy of Science, The Harry Ginzberg Memorial Prize of The University of Chicago, and the Hofheimer Prize of the American Psychiatric Association. Currently Dr. Dement is Professor of Psychiatry at the Stanford University Medical School.